Lighten Up!
7 Weeks to Release, Recharge and Revitalize!

Dr. Christina Tarantola, PharmD, CHC, CHt

Thank you to my parents, Maryann and Joe, for supporting me through it all. I am forever grateful for your generosity and the lessons I've learned through having you as my parents.

Thank you to my pharmacy contributor team –Marina, Nicole, Niloufar, Krissy, DawnDee, and the countless others who have contributed to the creation of this book.

Thank you to you, the reader, for being open to receive new ideas and concepts that will guide you to a new level in your life.

Table of Contents

Disclaimer

I am not a medical doctor, dietician, or nutritionist. I make no claims to cure, diagnose, or treat any disease. This book is meant to serve as an educational tool to guide you to feel empowered in your health. Please consult with your doctor if you have any questions about starting a new supplement, exercise, treatment or herbal regimen.

To the reader,

Lighten Up! is a step-by-step guide to supporting you in awakening to your fullest potential in your health. Throughout these 7 weeks, you will discover new techniques that will help you focus on your internal mindset and belief system to transform your physical health. What is equally as important as the food we are eating, is what we are feeding ourselves mentally, emotionally and spiritually. As you uncover and become aware of where you are getting in your own way, you will easily begin to align with health.

As you delve into this book, I want to encourage you to take your time reading through the material each week. Spend time focusing on the chapters within that week. Remember - this is a marathon, not a sprint! Whether you are looking to lose weight or have more energy, this book is meant to allow you to slowly unravel what no longer works in your life, leaving room for a renewed sense of aliveness. Don't feel you need to rush through the material!

Take your time. Take notes in a separate notebook and reflect. Complete the Weekly Reflections as this will help you integrate the concepts you've learned and deepen the process.

The purpose of this book is to awaken you to what has been holding you back in your health. The book is meant to help you uncover and let go of old beliefs, patterns, and stories that hold you back from living the vibrant life you deserve. Let's begin!

Preface

Just as a candle spreads light in a dark room, people who are living in their highest truth give off an energy that inspires everyone around them. Have you ever met someone like this? They emanate joy and "lightness" because they are connected to Spirit. People living in the light have the following qualities:

- They are excited about the work they do.
- They see the world as a friendly place.
- They at peace with themselves.
- They are kind rather than judgmental.
- They love to play.
- They are willing to be students as well as teachers.
- They are in awe of the world.
- They take great pleasure in serving others.

More often than not, these people are also healthy. If you are attuned to feeling the "vibe" or energy of others, it will feel extremely positive to be around these people. What is the secret to live in a space of joy and be full of light? Releasing old patterns, beliefs and ideas of who you've been conditioned to be and living in your most authentic truth allows you to be filled with light. Embodying the light means you are in alignment with who you really are. When you have these qualities you are automatically aligned with health. That is my goal for you as you read this book – to connect fully with your light and be a beacon for others in your world.

I have decided to create this book in response to many of my clients and friends asking how they could feel better, attract healthier relationships and start living the life of their dreams. We so often think to ourselves, "If only the _____ showed up, I would be happier." For you, maybe that "thing" is money, the man or woman of your dreams, a dream house or a fulfilling career. Whatever that is for you, you can have it when you are in touch with your "light."

When I look at my life today, it is much different than the quality of my life 6 years ago. I was not always a business owner, an author, or a person who even thought I could be or deserved to be happy. In fact, my core belief was "*I am not loveable,*" so I understand what it is like to struggle with self-doubt and fear. For many years I hid my true self in distractions, addictions, and relationships. I sought outside of myself in alcohol, cigarettes, food, and love to fill the wounds of my past, only to discover that things or people could never fill that emptiness. During that dark time, I was disconnected and depressed. I had been dimming my light, my essence, for so long that my life was not workable.

It took many years of suffering, being ashamed of who I was and dealing with anxiety, depression, and a rare eating disorder before I woke up to the fact that I was in need of healing.

My rock bottom was on March 29, 2012. I was kicked out of my home, jobless, and living out of my car. I can still visualize all of my belongings, coats with hangers still attached, shoes, makeup and clothes, laying sprawled out on my front lawn as my mother cursed and screamed from inside the house. Despite the chaos that surrounded me that day, I still had an overwhelming feeling that I was about to be transformed and that the old ways of being would not work any longer. With desperation in my voice, I said a prayer to God that if I ever healed and recovered, I would dedicate my life to serving humanity.

Well, if you haven't guessed, I did heal. What did it take? It took years of therapy, personal development seminars, reading books from the great works of Deepak Chopra, Melanie Beattie, Louise Hay, Dr. Wayne Dyer and countless others. When there is a problem that seems impossible to fix, you need to try everything you can at it until it is healed. The eating disorder lasted 7 long years, but I know the true healing came from the inner work I did. That is precisely what this book teaches.

Fast forward to today, I have studied nutrition, energy medicine, hypnotherapy, motivational interviewing and habit change, and how food can heal the body. After my transformation, I knew I needed not just to help people heal their body, but to also support their soul's growth.

My intention here is to empower you to take charge of your health so that you can shine more brightly in the world. When you set an intention to take care of yourself through radical self-love, you set a powerful example and create a domino effect in your family, community and in the world. Health is your foundation to do great work in the world, to take care of your family and experience joy, aliveness and fulfillment.

Ghandi said, "*Be the change you wish to see in the world*" and I can't help but believe that once you reclaim your health, you inspire others to do the same. I am so enthused and honored that you are here and I look forward to hearing how you've evolved and started this positive movement of "Lightening Up!"

What you'll need for this journey:

*If you are not a client and would simply like to read the book to learn more about health and healing, then you can skip this section! If you are a client, read on!

- ➢ Food scale
- ➢ Scale to track your progress
- ➢ Tape measure for your waist circumference
- ➢ Journal to track your journey, progress and food/exercise

> ➢ Download the MyFitnessPal app

Some other tips as you start:

1. **Have an authentic conversation with your family** and share about this new journey you are on. Studies show that people who have more support are more likely to succeed in their endeavors. There are no rules for this conversation, but I encourage you to enroll others in your goal pursuit! This will help you have an accountability team and an encouraging environment where you can flourish!

2. **Feel free to go at your own pace in this book.** If you find you want to digest (no pun intended!) the material, take your time. I do encourage you to write your answers to the Weekly Reflection in a journal so we can review the answers together in our weekly sessions.

3. **Be coachable.** It isn't always easy to look at ourselves, but please know that there is no judgment here. I am here as a member of your support system, cheering you along the entire way! I may ask you to try new techniques much like you would try on a new hat. If you don't like the hat, you do not have to wear it or buy it! Just try it on. I want you to find the tools that work best for you.

4. **Be honest and open.** As long as you tell the truth and are honest, you are on the right track. I don't expect you to lose 50 pounds in 2 weeks. My sole expectation is that you stay consistent with the material and stay open and honest with me! You'll do great!

Introduction

It is no coincidence that you are reading this book at this time in your life. However you came across it, the universe felt it was time for us to meet! I am grateful to share what I've learned over the past 6 years of coaching, guiding and assisting hundreds of people to discover - that long-term change comes from inner healing.

I believe that you are a soulful person, a genuine, caring and giving human being. I know you are someone who wants to feel better in your physical body. Maybe you have tried countless things to help you lose weight, and feel energized and confident in your body. In our society, the quick fix or the next best diet is commonplace. You may be someone who has said, "I've tried everything!"

I have learned that it isn't enough to use topical, temporary solutions. Shakes, supplements, prescription weight loss pills and skinny wraps don't fix the problem. Without looking at the cause, there can never be permanent change. Transformation is an inside job. To *transform* means to change form, which happens from within.

Your own personal journey will be different than your husband, wife, children, neighbor, and anyone else in your community. You have your own unique genetic makeup, schedule, food preferences, body type and maybe even food allergies or intolerances.

It can be tempting to look at your neighbor who lost 50 pounds from the ketogenic diet and not want to try it too! However, I encourage you to always follow your inner guidance and trust the wisdom of your own body.

Throughout this book, you may find that you release old concepts of what it takes to lose weight and be healthy. You may have picked up various beliefs from the internet, Dr. Oz or any other book, radio or t.v.

show. I encourage you to stick with what makes sense for *your unique health situation.* I am also willing to bet you will close this book with a better understanding of what works for you and have a compelling, exciting vision for your future health.

I will be sharing the powerful insights I have gleaned about weight loss and healing from personal experience and from working with countless incredible coaching clients. I have come to understand that there are certain patterns people exhibit when they are sick, overweight and energetically "heavy." When we "lighten" up physically, mentally, emotionally and spiritually, healing and health is automatically the result.

My own personal journey of going through anxiety, depression and two different eating disorders sparked a tremendous desire to help people heal their body through nutrition, behavior modification coaching, and hypnotherapy. This is my *why* and is what motivates me every day to write, speak and encourage people to heal.

I believe we all have a purpose here and if we are suppressing, denying and avoiding parts of ourselves or our past, we cannot move powerfully into the future. If we are not stepping into our light, our true divine nature, we cannot be healthy.

My goal in writing this book is to help guide you along a journey to healing. Not just in a physical sense but in a holistic way of you returning to wholeness. May you discover your light and be open to the next phase of your spiritual journey...

Week 1: Where True Healing Starts

Why We Get Sick

To "heal" means to make whole again. We are born perfect, whole and complete. Our parents and teachers mean well and share their beliefs freely in our innocent minds. From birth to 6 years old, children take in and believe whatever they are told. Children are eager and receptive to new ideas and cannot decipher for themselves what is "true" or "false."

Ideas like, *"Good girls don't behave that way"* or *"Little boys don't cry"* are common in many households. After all, our caretakers feed, clothe and shelter us and we want to make them happy! A child will conform to his or her family to remain safe. Perhaps when they tried to express themselves, they were suppressed or told to keep quiet. The more a child suppresses who they naturally are, the more they turn away from that perfect, whole and completeness that they are!

We carry many beliefs embedded in childhood into adulthood, which has a huge impact. We carry beliefs about our self-image, health, what is "normal", preconceptions about diseases our parents have, fears they have about money, politics, religion and so on. Those beliefs drive our actions as adults. By the time we grow up, most of these beliefs are *subconscious* or under the surface of our everyday actions.

When we suppress and deny aspects of who we are and avoid

feeling our emotions, we get sick. Our mental-emotional body is intimately connected to our physical body and when we keep stuffing down our emotions, what happens? We explode at some innocent bank teller or maybe we turn that guilt inward and silently suffer through numbing ourselves with food, alcohol, drugs, sex or gambling.

Emotions are energy in motion, and when that energy gets suppressed, it needs to go somewhere. The Diathesis-Stress Model states that human beings have a proclivity for certain illnesses due to our genetics and family history. When continued *stress* is applied to the body, the disease comes about physically. Stress can come from trauma (emotional or physical), toxins (chemical or environmental) or thoughts (mental and emotional.) Instead of resisting, suppressing or avoiding our emotions, simply being a witness to them allows the feeling to be released.

The fundamental aspects of health are many we know about – good nutrition, sleep, stress management, and movement. These "pillars" are the foundation of your physical "house" or body. When you do not have a strong foundation for your house, what happens? It breaks down, things fall apart, or the roof may spring a leak and so on. Keeping your physical body strong is important and will prevent 90% of disease!

Dis-ease, or a lack of harmony and balance in the body, manifests in many ways—from pain, headaches, anxiety, depression, fatigue, and acne, all the way to cancer. And we are all susceptible to it. There are many physical causes of disease as modern science has studied and documented. Smoking, excess consumption of animal meat and alcohol, lack of exercise, and both mental and physical stress are some causes, to name a few. Researchers have spent copious amounts of time and money to draw massive cohorts of people together to study, research, and document patterns of behavior, how the body responds to stress, and how to prevent and treat disease. Much of this research has helped create treatment algorithms that medical doctors now implement.

As a pharmacist, I have personally witnessed the miraculous workings of pharmaceuticals, which rescue millions of lives each year. Antiarrhythmic drugs help reestablish normal heart rhythms in patients with atrial fibrillation. Emergency-room doctors administer vasopressor, epinephrine, and other blood pressure stabilizers that literally save people's lives. I have also seen thousands of patients on opioids, mood-stabilizing medications, amphetamines, and appetite suppressants. These controlled substances leave a person tolerant, needing higher doses to achieve the same effect over time. Even many people on blood pressure medication were not satisfied with the adverse effects of their medications and wanted alternative answers. However, most medication is a Catch-22, a double-edged sword. First, you are only treating the "symptoms" and never getting to the root "cause." Also, your body is succumbed to a multitude of adverse effects including vitamin depletion and begins to rely on the medication to function.

As I began my work as a pharmacist, I became intimately involved with talking to patients about their experiences with medication as it related to their health condition. As I mentioned, most of them did not want to be on medication; they wanted a natural therapy. Many of them took vitamins, supplements, and over-the-counter products. They often asked their friends about their health conditions or even searched their symptoms on the Internet before going to a doctor. People wanted to feel better, to alleviate pain or lose weight or lower their blood pressure through natural means. That was the point when I realized that understanding pharmaceuticals alone would not serve my patients. I began learning more about alternative medicine, the healing benefits of food, and eventually energy healing and Applied Kinesiology.

Because of my own eating disorder and seeing so many sick patients coming back to the pharmacy month after month for refills and never improving, I became obsessed with understanding why people got sick and how they could heal. I searched for the answers in self-help books, sought out reading material from mind-body-medicine gurus like Dr. Deepak Chopra and Dr. Andrew Weil. Some of the most significant findings I came across were those of Barbara Brennan, who studied the tenets of energy healing, and Dr. David Hawkins, who studied Applied Kinesiology and calibrated the Energy Vibration Scale after 20 years of research.

Hawkins' research drew upon thousands of people over several decades, and his aim was to study kinesiology, how the body responded to false and true beliefs. He studied Electromagnetic Frequency (EMF), outlining a consciousness scale ranging from 0 to 1000. **See Figure 1 Scale of Consciousness.** False statements or harmful substances would weaken the person's muscles and lead to a strong emotional "No" reaction, whereas when a person held a life-promoting substance or spoke a true statement, their energy field was strengthened.

Thoughts such as guilt, shame, and fear kept people in a contracted, limited state, while love, joy, and gratitude led them to align with health and happiness. See the diagram below of the Scale of Consciousness. People who calibrate under level 200 (Courage) were found to have self-destructive behaviors like smoking, binge eating and lived in a state of fear. Those who calibrated above 200 behaved in self-promoting ways and were healthy.

The average level of consciousness (LOC) of the people in the United States calibrates around 200. However, someone at the level of Love (500) or above can raise the energy of 750,000 people below the level of 200. Someone at the level of Willingness can counter-balance

90,000 people below 200. Just by raising your own energy vibration, you can raise and lift others, many of whom you will never meet.

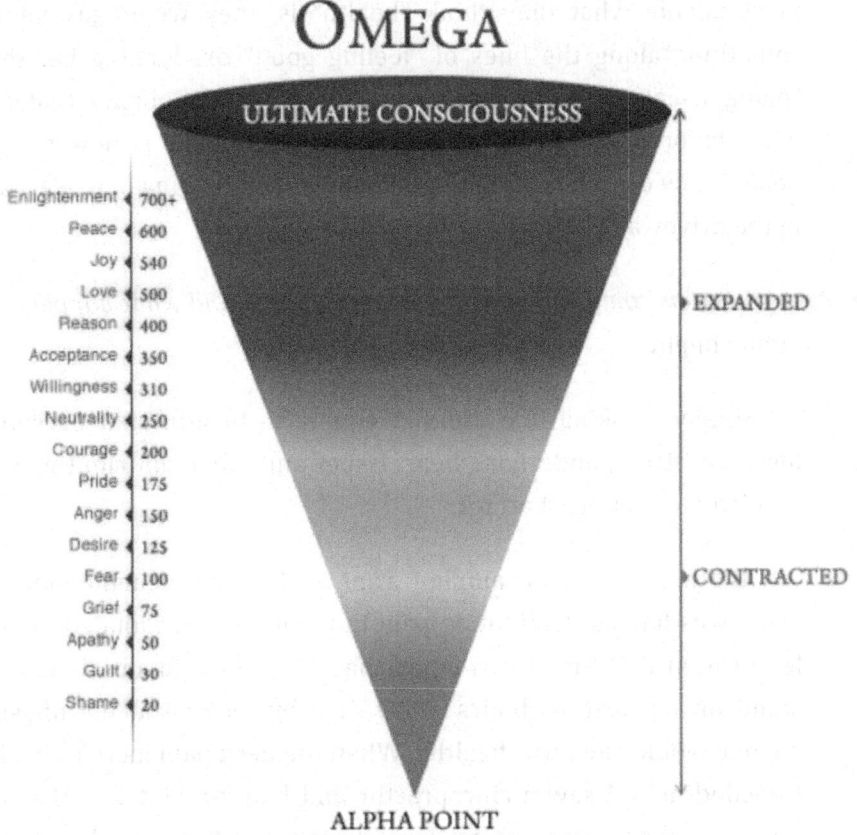

Figure 1. Scale of Consciousness

These patterns were correlated with what I began noticing with my clients. I saw many clients with diabetes and eating challenges, but the conversation was rarely just about food. Feelings of self-hatred, guilt, shame, anger, unwillingness to forgive, frustration, and other heavy emotions would surface as we worked through why they overate or tried to control their food. I realized then that people had certain energy blockages that prevented them from being healthy. The goal is to release and clear those old beliefs and patterns to move up the scale of consciousness.

Most of society doesn't view health this way. If you were to ask most people what they think "health" is, they would probably say something along the lines of "feeling good" or "looking healthy" or "being disease-free." Americans tend to look at the outside to decipher whether or not someone is healthy. If the outside is how we gauge health, how do you explain the 50-year-old man dying of a heart attack in the driveway?

"He was completely healthy. I don't understand what happened," his family might say.

Simply "looking fine" doesn't equate to health. That person may have had stress, underlying heart issues and other contributing factors that lead to that heart attack.

Another personal example I want to share happened about a year ago. I was having debilitating pain in my neck that radiated down my left arm. At that time I was a pharmacist working in a retail store and stood on my feet 10 hours a day. Just by looking at me physically, anyone would say I was healthy. When the neck pain increased, I knew I needed help. I saw a chiropractor and had x-rays taken that week. The normal curvature of the neck is supposed to be...well, curved. My neck was straight. After years of looking down at a pharmacy counter checking prescriptions, I was on the path to arthritis and permanent neck pain.

There is silent damage that occurs inside the body, and we cannot deny that health is more than just the "look good, feel good" mentality. We need to take our blinders off and see that health involves more than just putting a band-aid on a symptom or thinking we are healthy because nothing hurts today.

Health involves many pillars, including:
1. Proper nutrition
2. Movement
3. Mindfulness
4. Self-Care
5. Social Connections
6. Stress (Chemical, Emotional, Environmental)

When one or more of these components is off, the body starts to break down. Whether we can see the damage or not, the body is effected, and over time, disease will manifest.

Now I am not here to try to *scare you* but to put into perspective the way we tend to think. Throughout this book, your levels of awareness will increase, and you will become more in tune with your surroundings, including your body and how you treat it.

Now I mentioned before that I was not always a health coach or a healthy person. In 2012 many of those pillars listed above were out of balance.

1. **Nutrition** - I would be rigid and restrictive with my food during the day, only eating salads and "healthy foods" and then proceed to wake up at night and binge on cookies, cake, bread and peanut butter. This caused me daily anxiety and stress that would continue every single night for 7 years.

2. **Movement** - I was abusing my body and over-exercising to compensate for the extra calories I felt guilty about consuming.

3. **Mindfulness** – Yes, my mind was FULL...of limiting beliefs! My level of awareness was nil compared to what I know

now. I had never meditated or took time to be still.

4. **Self-Care** - I bet you don't have to guess this one. My level of self-care was at a 1 or 2 out of 10 at best.

5. **Social Connections** - I was isolated from my family and lived in isolation in an apartment in Queens. As a result, I became depressed.

6. **Stress** - I was smoking (chemical) and had past traumas (emotional) I had not yet dealt with or processed. I also worked 70-hour weeks at my residency.

As you can see, I was not the ideal picture of health. Yet, today each and every one of those factors has turned around. Of course, it did not happen overnight, and it wasn't easy. What in life is worth it and comes easy? Not many things I could think of! I had to look at aspects of my life that I had hidden and tucked away. I had to face parts of myself that I hated and denied. Yet, I am grateful that those trying times happened because it propelled me to dedicate my life to this work.

If you are going through a chaotic time, I hope to be a beacon of light for you. Everything is temporary, and you will get through this! You have survived 100% of your worst days, and this is your fresh start.

I became passionate about helping people heal because of my journey and seeing people come back to the pharmacy without their conditions improving. I started off as a pharmacist, a professional meant to dispense powerful medications to alleviate symptoms or pain. It seemed like the entire Tarantola family was meant to be pharmacists. My father, sister, uncle and aunt were all pharmacists too. I guess you could say it was in my DNA!

All throughout pharmacy school I learned how the body functioned normally, how people became sick and the mechanism of how pharmaceuticals worked to artificially and temporarily alleviate symptoms. Yet, when I tried to understand my eating disorder, the cause did not make sense. Why did I have this rare eating disorder and why was it so hard to stop it?

I became obsessed with understanding the deeper reason why people became sick and how they could heal. I studied work from Barbara Brennan, David Hawkins, Dr. Masuro Emoto and other mind-body gurus. Ultimately, my research left me with a few essential keys about disease.

Now don't worry - I am not going to throw a bunch of terms at you without data and science to back it up. I also won't overload you with overly complicated terms. However, I will be discussing a lot about "energy" in the context of vibrational energy fields. This may be the first time you are hearing about these concepts, so I encourage you to be open-minded! Quantum physics backs this up!

What I have discovered about healing and disease:

1. **Disease starts in the spiritual realm**, not the physical, like many of us assume. There are certain energetic patterns that start the disease process, which then lead to mental thoughts and finally physical symptoms. Spiritually, or better put, energetically, a person becomes disconnected from who they really are. In other words, they lose sight of who they are and instead get inundated with fears and limiting beliefs from their environment.

   If that goes on long enough, they start to have certain beliefs about themselves. The limiting belief of "*I am not enough*" is one that almost all human beings have. People will go to massive lengths to prove they are enough through achievements, degrees, and accolades. Depending on where there are energetic "kinks" in the body, dis-ease will begin to

9

manifest in that area physically. Imagine a hose with a kink in it. The water cannot flow easily just as energy cannot flow where there are energetic blockages. We will go over this in **Week 7 Understanding Your Personal Energy System**.

2. **In order to heal anything, you need to change the energy first.** If you try to address disease topically by utilizing only physical means such as medication, you will not heal. Simply addressing physical aspects will not heal or create lasting change. Shifting your energy state will help you heal.

   For example, stress has a feeling or an energy to it. Stress is tense, heavy, contracted and closed. When you feel "stressed," don't you usually have tension somewhere in your body? We already know that constant stress creates physical disease such as high blood pressure, anxiety and so on. As you will learn in a later chapter, stress is actually an internal state, which you have control over. Shifting how we relate to and take care of ourselves is imperative for healing.

3. **You must begin to see things better than they are in order to shift.** Tony Robbins talks about having a "compelling future vision" for your life. If you reinforce how horrible things are, guess what? They will continue to be horrible. What you constantly say to yourself internally will come about in the external world. Your words and thoughts also carry a frequency, and they can be disempowering or empowering. You must break the cycle at the level of thought and feeling in order to create a new reality for yourself.

With all of this talk about energy, I'd like to be clear about the title of this book. To "lighten up" means to begin releasing old "stuff" at the energetic level. We all carry beliefs, traumas and old emotional baggage in our energy field. For example, perhaps you've been holding onto a grudge or resentment against a family member for years. Maybe you have experienced heartbreak, loss, betrayal, and disappointment and haven't forgiven that person or forgiven yourself. All of your life experiences are there in your cellular DNA and releasing that "debris" opens the door for healing.

Many concepts in this book focus on releasing, letting go, surrendering and so on. That was an intentional design I had when I created this book! Every bit of what you will read is important and relevant to your health journey. Holding onto that pain literally weighs on you.

When you feel happy, you feel lighter don't you? If you think back to the happiest times in your life, I guarantee you weren't sick or overweight. You were probably loving life and felt energized!

My mission here is to help you release that heaviness that can stay stuck in your body unless looked at from an energetic standpoint. My goal is to help you step into your light as a fully embodied human being to enjoy life to the fullest. Notice the word enjoy means "in joy." At the level of joy, the body can heal itself. We will discuss more about this in the energy chapters.

Why Diets Don't Work

I went into Barnes and Noble recently and passed the dozens of shelves labeled "self-help." That is my favorite section! I love books on personal development. As I neared the health section, I noticed the countless books on diets. The Fast Diet, the DASH diet, the 10 Day Green Smoothie Cleanse. I was drowning in a sea of diets! Americans spend an average of $800 annually on diet supplements and products, including diet books promising to fix their weight issue.

We are always searching for the "quick fix" or the next best diet to try. Dieters tend to think thoughts like, "I'm not good enough" or "I'll be happy when I'm thin." The opposite is true!

You must realize that nothing outside of you will change how you feel on the inside. On the contrary, you must transform internally in order to see any outward change.

Let's explore....Why do most diets fail?

1. Many diets are *restrictive* and cut out certain food groups. For example, the Atkins diet and South Beach diet requires that you restrict carbohydrates for a certain period. This is not pleasant or sustainable. As you will learn in this book, each macronutrient (protein, carbohydrate, fat) has a role to play for your body. Our bodies are not designed to go on diets!

2. Most diets *force a person to rely on the pill, supplement, shake or product for a certain amount of time.* Why is the failure rate so high for dieters? Why do people regain the weight? Putting a band-aid over a problem will help it temporarily, but it won't solve the problem. Once that weight loss aid is removed, the weight slowly creeps back. Meal delivery systems give you meals, but what happens when your subscription is over, or when you go out to a party or out to eat with friends? There needs to also be flexibility.

3. Minimal or no focus on the *mindset component.* We are all going to have our stressful moments or times when we have little Johnny's birthday party. How will you plan for those events? Having awareness and anticipating possible barriers or challenges can help you work through them.

We know what *doesn't work.* Well, what does work, you might be asking?

Imagine someone asked you to build a shed. You'd need a hammer, nails and all of the other tools that my dad would know what to do with. The point is — you need tools, or knowledge, to be able to complete that project. The same goes for weight loss.

I hate to be the bearer of bad news, but….

There is no shortcut. There are no magic pills.

We must make the process fun and learn the principles to be able to translate it into long-term, weight loss.

The problem with the word "diet" is that it is a quick fix. This coaching program focuses on helping you create a permanent *lifestyle change.* Discovering what works best for your body may require support and knowledge about your specific medical history, food preferences, schedule, and goals. When you discover what works for you, you will feel more confident, energetic, and happy that you made a choice to take care of your body.

When you first start off on any journey, there is a lot of enthusiasm, excitement, and momentum. Think of how many people make resolutions on January 1st of each year. According to Forbes Magazine, 48% of Americans make a New Years resolution each year. Guess how many actually achieve their goal? Only 8%!

There are many reasons for this phenomenon – lack of self-regulation, unrealistic goals, an unsustainable plan and so on. When you set a powerful intention to change something in your life, everything that has been blocking you will come up to be recognized and cleared away. For example, many of my clients looking to lose weight have tried various diets, shakes, workout plans and failed at them. One reason they did not succeed was because of a lack of support and lack of practical tools that lead to permanent change.

I had a client who started his weight loss journey with me and lost 10 pounds in the first month. He was ecstatic! A month later, he had hit a plateau and felt frustrated. Upon a deeper look at the frustration, I realized that patience was something he struggled with. He was used to the instant gratification of getting what he wanted right away. As he examined his life, he saw that his lack of patience permeated his work, his home life and now his weight loss journey.

He was able to be curious about his patience, and through our coaching sessions, he discovered that he did have patience with certain activities. We were able to transfer those skills to his weight loss journey, and he began having less resistance and frustration.

We cannot always see what is tripping us up and preventing us from succeeding in our goal pursuit. In the case of my client, his lack of patience was a huge barrier to achieving his weight loss goals. He understood why his previous diet attempts had never worked! Without the full picture, it can often be difficult to shift.

When we just look at the surface or treat the physical symptoms, things will never change permanently. Think of the principle of homeostasis, or the tendency of the body to seek and maintain a condition of balance or equilibrium within its internal environment. The body is always going to come back to equilibrium. However, if you look at the root cause of why there is an imbalance, you can heal the problem.

You can have the best of intentions, but it takes discipline and resilience to achieve your goals. Life gets in the way. Maybe you have children, aging parents, a job and other responsibilities that require energy and attention. After some time, old patterns, excuses or forms of self-sabotage may creep in. You may be gung-ho in the beginning to get to your weight loss goals, but then one day it's raining out, and you don't feel like going to the gym. Perhaps you have to work late and wind up eating out of a box of Cheerios because you haven't planned for flexibility.

One of the first books I read by life and business strategist Tony Robbins was Awaken the Giant Within (Free Press, 1992). In that book, Tony writes about how human beings want to avoid pain and move toward pleasure. We do not want to repeat the past, and we fear failure in the future. As a result, we move away from anything that reminds us of a negative experience. I cannot help but think that the concept of pain and pleasure is a huge part of my work with clients who want to change their behavior.

We crave comfort and the familiar. It can be uncomfortable to change, especially when our past efforts have not been successful. Maybe you tried to lose weight and did not succeed. Perhaps you tried to start an exercise routine, but it did not stick. You might think it would be easier to make an excuse to avoid failing again.

Often we self-sabotage! Self-sabotage, also called self-handicapping, is when people do something that may thwart their performance in order to provide an excuse to explain subsequent failure.

Some examples of self-handicapping include procrastinating, delaying, distracting oneself with the internet, drugs or alcohol, and making excuses. We do this to avoid the anxiety and fear of facing ourselves and the issue at hand.

All these coping mechanisms lead to underachievement. If you self-handicap and fail at achieving a goal, you can blame the circumstances (procrastination or alcohol, for example). If you succeed, this increases your self-esteem, because you have done so despite challenging circumstances, and that gives you a boost.

We engage in this behavior because we want to stay safe and protected. Think about it: If you do not lose weight, you do not risk the possibility of being able to maintain it. The human brain wants to move away from pain and toward pleasure.

This coping mechanism can appear in all areas of life: career, relationships, health, and so on.

All of us have an internal voice that guides our actions. In other words, we talk to ourselves internally. *"It's OK if I miss my workout today because I ate pretty well,"* or, *"It is OK if I binged; I will exercise more."* These are called compensatory behaviors, and they undermine your goals.

As we form behaviors and ways of thinking, the patterns become ingrained in our neural pathways. Cognitive distortions are the catalyst for behaviors not in line with goals. For example, projecting, assuming, and predicting what that second slice of pie would taste like, *"That would taste really good; I need to have another slice,"* might be an internal conversation.

So how do we stop getting in our own way? We need to start talking to ourselves. Yes, I am suggesting you have internal conversations. The key is to notice your thoughts, reframe them and find constructive ways of coping. Behaviors do not just happen. They originate at the level of thought and emotion. If you can become aware of your thoughts and emotions, you can create a gap to choose before engaging in the old behavior.

Coaching can help guide you to discover what those internal conversations are and increase awareness around actively choosing and etching new pathways of habit. You will learn more about this in **Week 5: Finding Stillness in an Over-stimulated World.**

Reflection for Week 1:

1. What aspects of yourself do you love? What do you tend to hide or avoid about yourself?
2. What negative past experiences have shaped your view of your body and your health?
3. What are some of the limiting beliefs and self-talk you engage in?
4. Where and why does disease start?
5. What are the 6 pillars of health?

Week 2: Healing Through Nutrition

Food is Medicine

"Let medicine be thy food and let food be thy medicine."

– Hippocrates 400 B.C.

I used to see patients coming into the pharmacy every month for the same set of prescriptions. High blood pressure, high cholesterol, and diabetes medications were even timed on "auto-fill" so that those prescriptions would be filled on the same day each month. There was virtually no preventative strategy to get them OFF medication. No one questioned it. It was just standard procedure to keep prescription volume and profits up.

Something about that never sat quite right with me. When I started teaching diabetes classes at my Community Pharmacy Residency in Brooklyn, I saw a new pattern as I spoke to my patients. They didn't want to be on medication and wanted to lower their blood sugar through diet and exercise. In pharmacy school, we get one class on nutrition and a bare minimum of how to counsel patients on making lifestyle changes.

As I began reading more and taking online nutrition classes at The Institute for Integrative Nutrition, I realized that food is medicine. Each person is unique; their DNA, body type, metabolism, and food

17

preferences are different.

With each condition, there are various modalities of healing that can mitigate symptoms and improve overall health. For example, many studies have shown that having a mindfulness or yoga practice can improve Rheumatoid Arthritis symptoms. Balancing blood sugar and consuming more vegetables can help lower disease risk. There are countless natural ways to improve your health!

Food is medicine. The field of Nutrigenomics studies how food influences gene expressions and contributes to either health or to disease.

Nutrigenomics is based on several concepts:

- Genes play a role in disease development and prevention.
- A poor diet can be a serious risk factor for many diseases.
- Nutrient deficiencies and toxic chemicals in low-quality foods have an effect on human gene expressions.
- Each person is different regarding how much their diet impacts their genes/health.
- A healthy but also personalized diet can be used to prevent, mitigate or cure chronic diseases.

The food we eat can impact what proteins genes produce according to our DNA. Take caffeine as an example. Many people can drink caffeine and go to sleep 20 minutes later, while others cannot drink it after a certain time in the afternoon. We metabolize differently!

Just as some bodies react differently than the norm to certain foods, how people metabolize medications can vary as well. Pharmacogenomics looks at how drugs impact people based on how quickly they metabolize the drug. Prescription doses will depend on whether someone is a slow metabolizer or rapid metabolizer.

With Nutrigenomics, as doctors better understand how a patient's body handles nutrients and supplements, they'll be able to better predict the effects of a particular drug or a dosage without having to wait and see how the patient responds.

Each food has various properties that can enhance health. Carrots have beta-carotene and vitamin A, C, E that support eye health. Blueberries have anthocyanin, an antioxidant that benefits every cell in the body. Free radicals are harmful by-products of environmental toxins. Typically, atoms have pairs of electrons, but free radicals "steal" an electron, leaving that atom extremely unstable. Free radicals cause cell damage and contribute to aging and disease. Eating more antioxidant foods like blueberries, goji berries, dark chocolate, blackberries, and cilantro can help to counteract the damage done to cells.

Consuming whole foods is another way to improve your health. Taking a lycopene supplement will not give you the full range of additional vitamins, minerals, and fiber that a tomato would, for example.

Some of the top whole foods I recommend are:

1. **Berries.** My personal favorites are strawberries, blackberries, and raspberries. Berries have a high level of antioxidants, which help prevent free radical damage to cells. They can also be a great alternative to sugar when you are craving something sweet. Top your oatmeal, yogurt or cereal with berries.

2. **Cruciferous vegetables** like broccoli, cauliflower or brussel sprouts. Not only do these vegetables have fiber and vitamins, they have been shown to reduce the risk of certain cancers. I

chop up brussel sprouts, sprinkle chopped walnuts, dried cranberries, drizzle olive oil and bake them at 350 for 15-20 minutes. This is a great healthy option for dinner, holidays or parties.

3. **Ginger, garlic and green tea.** Not all together! These three foods have anti-inflammatory properties which help with conditions like arthritis, auto-immune conditions and even diabetes. Green tea has been shown to support weight management.

4. **Oatmeal.** I eat this for breakfast every day with a scoop of pea protein powder. Oatmeal helps keep you full and also has soluble fiber to promote cholesterol management. Top it with cinnamon powder, berries or a drizzle of manuka honey.

5. **Oily fish like salmon.** Full of omega 3 fatty acids, salmon, albacore tuna and sardines also support reduction in inflammation.

Utilizing food as medicine can improve health outcomes and support your body to work optimally. Be sure to include a wide variety of foods in your diet so that you are getting enough nutrients. See **Appendix B** of this book for ideas on healthy breakfast, lunch, dinner and snack recipes.

Are You Sabotaging Your Nutrition Efforts?

We have all heard, the phrase *"You are what you eat,"* but what counts the most? Quantity? Quality? Total number of calories? There is so much information out there on the internet; it can be confusing to sort through it all!

When it comes to a sustainable lifestyle change, there are many things to take into consideration such as food preferences, work/life schedule, body type and so on. However, there are a few key principles that impact everyone across the board.

Food is a key pleasure in our life! It is okay to use food to nourish your body *and* indulge every so often. I use the 80/20 rule, where 80% of my food comes from whole food sources and 20% is "fun food." Where we run into a problem is when we eat too much, too quickly and consume low quality food.

Here are three ways you may not realize you are sabotaging your healthy eating plan and the solutions to help!

1. **Eating too much** – Plain and simple - portion sizes that are too big. Going back for second and third helpings contributes to consuming extra calories. Repeat this enough, and you will gain weight. It takes 3500 excess calories to gain 1 pound.

Some people are "weekday dieters" and only follow their nutrition plan on the weekdays. They then go out on weekends and consume excess amounts of alcohol and ingest extra calories eating out at restaurants.

It's simple...

Calories consumed > calories burned = weight gain
Calories consumed < calories burned = weight loss

Solution:

a. Change your environment. If you take your food to the couch to eat and watch t.v., change it up! Be present and sit at a table.

b. Start measuring and weighing your food. Don't just guess that something weighs 3 ounces. Measure it! Fats like nuts or peanut butter are easy to estimate and go overboard on since fats are more calorie dense.

c.   If you are out at a restaurant and don't want to bring your handy-dandy scale, use the **MyPlateMethod. See Appendix B – Dinner** for the MyPlate diagram. This will help ensure you are getting a balanced meal.

Use a 9" plate and mentally divide the plate in half. Half of the plate should consist of leafy green vegetables or another non-starchy vegetable like carrots or string beans. The other half of the plate can mentally be divided in two. One-quarter of the plate will be a lean protein such as chicken, fish, turkey, tofu or another vegetarian option for protein. The other one-quarter will be a starchy carbohydrate like a sweet potato, brown rice or whole grain bread. Viola! You have your meal!

2. **Eating too quickly** - Eating while distracted. This could mean looking at your phone, being on your computer or on a phone call. Eating too quickly also means your brain doesn't have time to register to your stomach that it is full. This feeds back into number 1. Studies show that distracted eaters consume up to 50% more calories.

Solution:

a.   Put your fork down in between each bite. Do your best to chew your food 20 times before swallowing it. Chewing your food aids in digestion and metabolism.

b.   Put all electronics away and on silent or airplane mode. Be fully present with your meal. If you have a family dinner, have everyone put their phones in a basket until the meal is done. Distraction can cause you to consume more than you think.

3. **Eating low-quality food** - Continuously eating low quality, nutrient depleted food leads to poor health. Garbage in, garbage out. If you are eating poor quality food, you won't have energy! Limit processed foods such as baked goods, pretzels, candy and pretty much anything that has ingredients you can't pronounce.

Processed foods have more than 5 ingredients and the first one listed is the most concentrated in the product. Anything with less than 5 ingredients is minimally processed or a whole food source. Ingredients like high fructose corn syrup, MSG or food dyes are the more popular offenders that need to be avoided. Studies have shown a direct link between consumption of high fructose corn syrup and obesity. Also, opt for grass-fed beef, organic, hormone-free chicken as these options will have a higher nutrient value and less or no added hormones.

Whole food sources include anything found in nature such as vegetables, fruits, nuts, seeds, animal protein, grains, etc.

Solution:

a. Be aware of where your food is coming from and read Nutrition Labels. Even if a package "looks" healthy, always read the Nutrition Facts and the ingredient list. The more you are aware of the ingredients, calorie content or nutrient quality, the better decisions you can make to stay healthy.

b. Utilize the 80/20 rule. Twenty percent of your food can be from "fun foods" or anything that isn't a whole food source. It is about moderation, not deprivation!

Each food has an energy to it. Foods like vegetables, fruit, nuts, and seeds have a higher frequency than foods like meat, dairy, sugar and alcohol. When I say "higher frequency", I mean that, on a molecular level, those particles vibrate at a faster rate. The faster the rate, the lighter the particle. When people say, "I'm eating light today" and opt for a salad there is an actual science behind it! "Low-frequency foods" are composed of particles that vibrate at a slower rate and are thus heavier.

The Ancient Greeks believed that eating high-energy foods helps us reach higher states of consciousness and better connect with Source. This is one of the reasons many ancient philosophers and healers such as Plato and Pythagoras were vegetarians.

Some examples are organic fruits and vegetables, legumes, and nuts. Essentially, they come from the earth. Eating these types of foods results in health and harmony in the body, whereas foods with a low vibrational quality result in sickness and disharmony.

Food impacts your energy levels, mood and more obviously, weight. Consuming high-quality food is imperative for optimal health.

We can derive so many healing benefits from the foods we choose to consume each and every day. It is truly medicine, and we can choose to eat high-quality, nutrient-dense foods to prevent illness.

Examples of High Vibrational Foods:

- Wheatgrass
- Fresh certified organic fruit and vegetables
- Natural supplements such as spirulina
- Herbal Teas
- Herbs and spices
- Pure or filtered water
- Olive oil
- Nuts and seeds

- Fermented Foods
- Raw chocolate (cacao nuts or their butters)
- Raw honey & maple syrup
- Legumes
- Fermented foods
- Grains such as couscous, kamut, buckwheat, brown rice, amaranth, spelt and barley

What to expect from eating high vibrational foods:

When you initially start to eat these foods, you may experience the release of trapped emotions and changes in energy levels. Fatigue, headache or nausea may occur because of the body's natural detoxification process. Make sure you are drinking plenty of water and resting your body. Be gentle with yourself, especially if you are used to eating processed foods or low vibrational foods (See list below.) The way you eat will influence your mood and elevate your outlook on life because your vibrational energy is lifted.

It may also be helpful to write in your journal how you feel before and after you start incorporating these high vibrational foods in order to see the clear difference in energy state, mental clarity and how your body feels.

Examples of Low Vibrational Foods:

- Meat, poultry, and fish
- Genetically modified (GMO) food, and conventional food that has been treated with chemicals and pesticides
- White rice and flours
- Sugars and artificial sweeteners
- Coffee or caffeinated beverages
- Alcohol
- Processed, packaged, or canned foods

- Unhealthy oils like canola, cottonseed, margarine, lard and vegetable oils
- Frozen foods
- Pasteurized cow's milk, yogurt, and cheese
- Cooked foods, deep-fried foods and microwaving food

Also, the way you prepare the food will change the quality of it. Minimize use of microwaving as it changes the life energy of that food. Instead, you can bake or broil the food to heat it.

I have found that negative thought patterns and consuming too much sugar, caffeine, and "low quality" foods leads to weight gain, low energy, and even anxiety. We deserve to wake up feeling vibrant and alive! This starts in the physical form by nourishing your body.

As you begin to incorporate more high vibration foods, you will notice several things:

- You will begin to attract positive people in your life as the frequency of negative people will not match yours anymore.
- You may have a strong desire to help the world in some deep and meaningful way.
- You will feel light in your body and even a spontaneous sense of joy.
- You will realize that when people are reacting to you, they are really projecting their fears.
- You notice an enormous amount of compassion that manifests as an expansion in your heart for all creatures and the world in general.
- You nourish your body with healthy foods because it makes you feel energized, positive, and refreshed.
- Material things do not draw your attention anymore; instead, you focus on cultivating your dreams and ideas.

As you lighten up what you eat, you will automatically notice a shift in your physical energy and take the next step to optimal health!

Metabolism, Thermogenesis & Macronutrients oh my!

Now you know about food quality, but let's break down the top macronutrients: protein, carbohydrate, and fat. Why do we care about looking at these macronutrients?

Macronutrient breakdown is important as each component provides its own unique contribution to the nutrition equation. Knowing what each macronutrient is, examples of each and the function of the body will help you understand why you are structuring your meal plan this way.

Before we go into macronutrient components, we need to address how metabolism impacts your body and plays an important role in your progress. Metabolism is the rate at which food gets broken down and assimilated and used. Today Energy Expenditure is broken down into two parts - functional and basal metabolism. You may have heard of your Basal Metabolic Rate or BMR. This is your base metabolism at rest. If you just sat in the same spot all day, the amount of calories you would burn would be your BMR. BMR is only 60-70% of the total metabolism equation.

Total Energy Expenditure = Functional Metabolic Rate + Basal Metabolic Rate

Functional metabolism, on the other hand, is variable and depends on activity and the food you consume. Yes, food can actually increase your metabolic rate! Functional metabolism is 30-40% of total energy expenditure. That means that you can increase your metabolism by increasing exercise and consuming the right quantity and quality of food at the right times. If you are feeling hopeful, then stick with me! If you feel overwhelmed, take it one piece at a time.

You may be asking yourself, *"How can eating food increase my metabolism?"* Food actually creates heat in the body, otherwise known as thermogenesis. *Thermo* = heat, *genesis* = creation of. Each macronutrient has a different thermic potential, which simply means that each food creates a certain amount of heat. For example, protein has a thermic effect of around 30%, whereas fat has 0-5%.

A simple way you can look at this is to think of a time you went shopping for a shirt. Say it was $100 (you're at Banana Republic) and you had the option to get 5% off or 30% off the shirt. Which would you choose? Why? Most of us want the deeper discount to get a good bang for our buck! The same principle applies to macronutrients. Protein gives you a better bang for your buck, while fat has a significantly less "discount."

You can maximize your metabolism by taking advantage of food timing, quality (macronutrient composition) and quantity! Now that you have this information let's dive into the individual macronutrients.

Here are the fast facts about macronutrients:

Macronutrient	Protein	Carbohydrate	Fat
Calories per gram	4 calories per gram	4 calories per gram	9 calories per gram
Function of macronutrient	Builds and repairs muscle and other cells; can reduce the effects of cortisol	With adequate protein consumption, increases metabolism and muscle growth; excess can be stored as body fat	Keeps you full, builds hormones, helps brain health
Thermic effect	20-30% thermic effect	5-30% thermic effect	0-5% thermic effect
Composition	Made of amino acids	Made of glucose	Made of fatty acids

Protein

Protein is important for boosting metabolism and is the building block for muscle growth. Proteins are long chain amino acids, which comprise foods like meats, dairy products and to a lesser extent, plant foods like beans and seeds. Eating too little protein can result in a sluggish metabolism, low energy, and trouble losing weight. Eating too much protein can impact your kidney function and does not have any benefit above the upper limit for your protein requirement. Calories are calories, and even if you eat extra protein, you will store those calories which will be stored as fat.

Examples of protein sources:

- Meat (turkey, chicken, beef, pork)
- Fish (salmon, tilapia, tuna)
- Beans (garbanzo, black beans)
- Legumes (lentils)
- Seeds (flaxseed, chia seeds)
- Vegetables (spinach, kale, brussel sprouts)

- Grains (quinoa, oats, buckwheat, amarynth)
- Protein powders (collagen, bone broth)

Carbohydrates

I cannot tell you how many people ask me about the ketogenic diet, Atkins, South Beach and all of these "low carb" diets. Carbs are not the devil, I promise!!

Carbohydrates are important for anabolism or muscle building. There have been many misconceptions about carbohydrates, and many people are afraid of carbohydrates because of the years of conditioning from the media, friends, and family. These fears are far from the truth!

Certain types of carbohydrates actually have a high thermic potential, even up to 30%! Complex carbohydrates, or those that are more slowly digested like sweet potatoes or spinach, are examples. Now you know why typical diets are high in protein and salads! They create the most heat to fuel your metabolism!!

Simple carbohydrates, or foods that cause an insulin spike due to the high glycemic load, have a lower thermic effect of 5%. Examples include sugary foods like donuts, pastries, cookies, pretzels or many other packaged foods.

Where most people get in trouble is when they decrease carbohydrates over a span of two months or more. You actually *decrease* your metabolism by UP TO 50% when you do this. It makes sense, right? You don't create as much heat when you do this, and your metabolism slows. *Slowly* increasing the amount of carbohydrates you consume will help you restore your metabolism.

Examples of carbohydrates include:

Starchy carbohydrates:
- Sweet potatoes
- Brown rice
- Whole grain bread
- Buckwheat
- Bulgur
- Quinoa
- Millet

Non-starchy carbohydrates:
- Carrots
- Broccoli
- Kale
- Spinach
- Collards
- Cauliflower
- Peppers

Non-starchy carbohydrates provide plenty of fiber to improve gastrointestinal motility and keep you full. Soluble fiber is "soluble" in water. When mixed with water it forms a gel-like substance and swells. Soluble fiber has many benefits, including moderating blood glucose levels and lowering cholesterol. Good sources of soluble fiber include oats and oatmeal, legumes, barley, fruits and vegetables.

Insoluble fiber does not absorb or dissolve in water. It passes through our digestive system in close to its original form. Insoluble fiber offers many benefits to intestinal health, including a reduction in the risk and occurrence of constipation. Most of insoluble fibers come from the bran layers of cereal grains.

Fat

Fat is the most calorie dense of the macronutrients at 9 calories per gram. Even though fat has the lowest thermic potential of all of the macronutrients, it is still needed for many bodily functions. Cutting fat down too low can result in hormone disruption and vitamin deficiency. Fats are needed for production of hormones, to coat the myelin sheath of nerve cells in the brain and provide the feeling of fullness. Fats also help absorb fat-soluble vitamins like vitamin A, D, K and E.

Examples of Fat include:

- Oils (olive, coconut, avocado)
- Avocado
- Coconuts
- Chia or flaxseed
- Ghee
- Nut butter (peanut, almond, cashew)
- Nuts

As a recap:

- ➤ Total Energy Expenditure = Basal 60-70% + Functional Metabolism 30-40%.
- ➤ Each macronutrient has a certain thermic potential that can be utilized to maximize your metabolism.
- ➤ Protein has a thermic effect of 20-30% and helps the body build and repair cells.
- ➤ Carbohydrates have a thermic effect of 5-30% and help the body gain muscle and maintain a robust metabolism.
- ➤ Fats have a thermic effect of 0-5% and provide a feeling of fullness along with production of hormones, and coat the myelin sheath of nerve cells in the brain.

For more guidance around meal structuring, see **Appendix B**, Healing Through Nutrition Menu of Breakfast, Lunch, Dinner and Snack Recipes.

Reflection for Week 2:

1. Write a list of the foods you enjoy eating from the high vibration foods list. You can use this as you build your next grocery list.

2. Fold a blank sheet of paper in half. Write out on a sheet of paper the following:

Fill in the right column with foods you enjoy eating that fit into the macronutrient category for that meal. Ex: Breakfast is protein/carbohydrate. You could write oatmeal and protein powder as an example. This is helping you build your own meal plan.

Breakfast	
Lunch	
Dinner	
Snack	
Pre-workout / Post workout	

Write out three examples of low quality foods.

a. _____

b. _____

c. _____

Week 3: Getting In Tune With Your Body

Bringing Awareness to Your Physical Body

So many of us are "in our heads" worrying about paying bills, picking kids up from school and living our daily lives that we are disconnected from our body. Cultivating awareness of your body is important to prevent burnout and lower your risk of stress-related illnesses.

Body awareness involves many aspects including noticing when we are stressed, hungry, tired and our body is telling us something. Often we are so busy that we ignore the signs our body gives us. For example, if you get a headache, you may take a pain relief pill. You could be getting headaches from dehydration, stress or any number of factors. Becoming more in tune with your body in all aspects will help you identify when you are out of balance and allow you to restore your well-being.

There is a reason medical professionals say, *"Stress is the silent killer."* We don't always feel high blood pressure or the effects of stress like neck tension right away. Signs and symptoms of stress include shallow breathing, headaches, fatigue, muscle spasm, insomnia and the list goes on. However, if we work at the source of stress, we can have control over it.

What I'd like you to do this week is to notice where you hold your stress. Is it in your stomach? Your neck? Are you tensing your shoulders or having shallow breathing? Set a timer on your phone twice a day to do a body-scan check-in. Ask yourself, "What do I need at this moment?" And don't say a martini! What is your body craving? Movement? Water? A snack?

Instead of reflexively going for your normal pattern, try something different. Give your body what it needs at that moment. The more you can detect early signs of stress or any other sensation, the more you will know your body and take the best care of it.

As you begin to bring more awareness to your body, it will feel natural to you to also eat more mindfully and gauge your hunger level. A useful tool I encourage clients to utilize is called the Appetite Scale. It is a scale from 1 to 10 that allows you to see how hungry you are before you eat. At a level 1, you are not hungry at all. You could look at a pizza and not want anything. At a level 10, you are starving and would eat pretty much anything.

I encourage you to develop your own Appetite Scale and see at what level you might need a snack or a meal. Maybe for you, a 5 indicates you need a snack and an 8 means you need a meal. Each person is different. Start noticing your hunger levels during the day. This will also show you where you may need a snack or to have a bigger meal. Ex: If you always feel hungry at 10:30 and you eat a light breakfast at 9 you can either add more to your breakfast or realize you need to have a snack at that 10:30 time.

In addition to getting in tune with your body, it is important to examine potential barriers that may creep up on your journey and prevent you from reaching your goals. Some of those barriers may be internal or external.

Internal barriers may include negative self-talk, cognitive distortions (see **Week 4: Overcoming Resistance**), fears and limiting beliefs. A limiting belief is a thought you hold in your conscious or subconscious mind that holds you back from reaching your goal. For example, fear can stop someone from taking action on something they need. I did this myself! I avoided making an appointment with the dentist when I knew I needed my wisdom teeth pulled. Why did I do that? I was afraid!

The opposite to fear is action. I encourage you to reframe your fear and instead create excitement around that fear. Unlike popular belief, fear is simply an indicator to keep moving forward. Think of a time when you were afraid of doing something. Do you remember the first time you rode your bike or went swimming swimming in a deep body of water? You were scared! Yet, you realized that you could do it! Fear is internal.

On the other hand, there are external barriers that may sabotage you. If your goal is to try to lose weight, those external barriers could be:

➢ Being around "trigger foods" at parties, restaurants or business functions.
➢ Distractions like t.v., texting, emailing, reading, cleaning or doing anything else to avoid exercising, planning out your meals or doing some other activity related to your goal. This is similar to procrastinating.
➢ Being "too busy" or making excuses to avoid being present with your priorities.

Certain "trigger" foods can cause you to slide back to old patterns. For me, peanut butter was a huge trigger food for my night eating. I could not keep peanut butter in the house because I felt out of control and would eat a large portion of it.

Eating behaviors are impacted by psychological factors like anxiety, depression, distorted body image, and perfectionism. Lacking the ability to identify and manage tough emotions impacts food behaviors.

Willpower alone will not lead to change. Willpower is part of the conscious mind and is only 5-10% of our total awareness. The "What the Hell Effect" is a real phenomenon! Have you ever opened a box of Girl Scout cookies, ate two cookies and said, "Eh- What the hell?" and polished off an entire sleeve...or box? That is the "What the Hell Effect" at play.

Overcoming this phenomenon requires looking at how you deal with setbacks. Do you automatically shift to self-criticism and beat yourself up? The trick is to shift into self-compassion instead, which may seem counterintuitive! You may be saying, "*If I am not hard on myself, I'll slip up!*" This is exactly opposite of what is true. Being compassionate with yourself turns off the guilt and prevents a second binge episode.

In one study (Adams, 2007), researchers asked a group of women to eat a doughnut within four minutes, then drink a glass of water so they would feel full. After eating the doughnut, some of the women received a message of self-compassion encouraging them to not be so hard on themselves for indulging. The other group did not receive this message.

In the second part of the study, the women were presented with bowls of candy and were invited to eat as little or as much of the candy as they wanted. The women who had received the self-forgiveness message ate only 28 grams of candy compared to the 70 grams consumed by the group that didn't get the message. That's a big difference!

If and when you find yourself in a situation where you have over-indulged, ask yourself the following questions:

1. What am I saying to myself? Am I being self-critical?
2. What would I say to a friend who had this happen?
3. Where do I have control or influence in this situation? This activates a can-do mindset, which has been linked to higher levels of well-being and health.

By shifting your perspective and being in tune with yourself, you can overcome potential barriers that may thwart your efforts.

Breaking the Cycle of Food Addiction

Many people are addicted to food and may not be aware that they are numbing their emotions by using food. I shy away from such terms as "emotional eaters" to avoid labeling anyone as having a 'dis-ease' or disorder. You are much more than a label or a behavior. You are a beautiful, feeling human being. However, many people eat when they are emotional. Stress, anger, frustration, guilt, and many other emotions can trigger a binge. The way to become more aware of this pattern is to not dissociate from your feelings.

Dissociating from your emotions happens when you "step outside of yourself" and disconnect from yourself. It is too painful to feel those feelings, so you dissociate. Trauma typically precedes dissociation and can stem from psychological, sexual, or physical abuse.

What is a "trauma?" If some event in your life produced an intense emotional response, it is a trauma. Do not minimize what happened to you, even if it's small compared to other people. I have heard many people say, *"Well, I have no right to complain about my father ignoring me or verbally abusing me. There are people out there who have been sexually abused."* If it's relevant and significant to you, then it was traumatic.

When I had my eating disorder, I used food as my crutch. I would deprive myself during the day and stay rigid in how I ate, portioning everything out perfectly. Then when I came home at night, I would binge on cookies and cereal in shame. It was all or nothing. There was no middle ground where I would allow myself to be in touch with what I really wanted or needed.

What is Food Addiction?

1. Compulsive overeating that triggers intense pleasure and leads to a reward.
2. Normal signals of satiety are overridden, and a person feels preoccupied with food or exercising to compensate for increased caloric intake.
3. Continue to eat despite negative consequences (weight gain or impacting relationships).
4. A loss of control to stop eating certain foods.

Food addiction is both chemical and emotional. I used food to numb, heavy emotions like loneliness, pain, and anger, and to fill the emptiness I felt. Often, binge eating quells those feelings because of a chemical response from the brain as well as the temporary feeling of fullness that follows.

Self-medication with food to ease tension, depression, or anxiety is common, and most people with this pattern have similar sensations that are likened to drug withdrawal. When you take away the substance, the body feels the effects, just like a coming off of a drug. You may feel headache, nausea, and strong mood changes. Racing thoughts trigger emotions, which trigger overeating. Lessening the heavy emotions and learning to cope is how you begin to overcome emotional eating.

How do you know you're addicted to food?

Do you:

- End up eating more than planned when you start eating certain foods?
- Keep eating certain foods even if you're no longer hungry?
- Eat to the point of feeling ill?
- Worry about not eating certain types of foods or worry about cutting down on certain types of foods?
- When certain foods aren't available, go out of your way to obtain them?

Other signs include:

- Hiding unhealthy food that you've eaten from others.
- Getting cravings for certain foods even after you've eaten a nutritious meal and feel full.
- You have repeatedly tried to set rules about certain foods but have been unsuccessful.
- Having withdrawal effects when stopping certain foods.

Food addiction can lead to isolation from friends and family, avoiding professional situations involving food and problems functioning at work or school. Also, food addiction can lead to depression, anxiety, low self-esteem and emotional numbness.

Food addiction is caused from a few sources. Our food supply, increasing stress levels and lack of emotional coping mechanisms are a few of those causes. Americans have the most overweight citizens in the world. I cannot help but think that it is the hydrogenated oil, high fructose corn syrup, and chemically modified food in the bulk of what we consume. Many are not aware that McDonald's and other fast-food chains submerge their fries and burgers in food additives that increase a person's craving for the food. Many foods and beverages such as soda, breads, ketchup, and cereals have high fructose corn syrup, which alters satiety hormones that tell your brain when you're full. These chemicals increase appetite and lead to weight gain and insulin resistance.

The power of choice and what food/beverages we put into our bodies is dependent on so many things—taste, convenience, and a physiological response to food additives that increase cravings for certain foods.

Researchers have done MRIs on the human brain after the subject ate a candy bar and the same area of the brain lit up as that of a person who was on cocaine. Eating a sweet piece of chocolate triggers intense feelings and memories about pleasure as well as activating dopamine receptors in the brain. These feelings originate from the dopamine reward system. (Dopamine is a neurochemical that regulates motivation, pleasure, and reinforcement related to certain stimuli—such as food.) The amount of pleasure we derive from eating a food correlates with the amount of dopamine released in the brain.

Also, neuroimaging has been done to prove that obese individuals have a less sensitive response to dopamine due to a down-regulation of receptors in the brain. This means there are less receptor sites for dopamine, which is why an obese individual needs more of the substance (food) to achieve the effect (pleasure). It will take an obese person a higher quantity of food to feel the effects of fullness and pleasure. They have a greater desire for food with a diminished reward response. This is why many people have sugar cravings that cannot be quelled by a single handful of M&Ms.

I have found several powerful tools to increase awareness and create leverage to choose healthy foods. Some are related directly to food and others are mental/emotional/spiritual tools. I will discuss all of these, so you feel empowered to take control of your life. You may feel hopeless when you are constantly in a cycle of food addiction or numbing your feelings. There is a solution.

The first tool you can utilize is to keep a food log of how you feel with each food you eat immediately after you eat it, then one hour after. Write down how your body feels, your level of energy from 0 to 10, and how your mood is affected. Certain people are intolerant to gluten, dairy, or caffeine. You may have been so busy throughout your day that you did not even pay attention to how food affected your energy and mood.

Logging your food and writing down how you feel afterwards will serve two purposes. First, you will become mindful of everything you are eating and drinking. Doing this may surprise you! You may notice you are continuously noshing throughout the day, grabbing a handful of your kids' fries or drinking more soda than you thought. The second function it serves is connecting what you eat to how your body feels. This is different than how your mind perceives the food. If you connect what you eat with how you feel, you will naturally want to choose more healthful foods.

Another helpful way to decrease cravings for sugar is to implement fermented foods into your diet. Fermented foods are carbohydrate-based and have had time to ferment, or allow good bacteria to germinate and therefore colonize your gut. These foods are typically low in calories and can help decreasing cravings for sugar.

Fermented foods:

1. Sauerkraut – I like Trader Joe's Sauerkraut with Persian cucumbers.
   How to consume it: Use sauerkraut on chicken sausage or top it onto any meat dish.

2. Kombucha – Kombucha is a bubbly, typically flavored drink loaded with B vitamins, minerals and strains of probiotic cultures. I like GT's Enlightened Kombucha since the sugar content is relatively low and it is inexpensive compared to other brands.

    How to consume it: Drink daily.

3. Pickles – Mostly anything pickled will have been fermented. In this case, cucumbers are pickled until they ferment.

    How to consume it: Top pickles on a salad or have as a side with your meal.

For more information on maintaining a healthy Gastrointestinal Tract (GIT) see **Appendix A.**

Ensuring you have plenty of protein and fiber in your diet is another way to decrease cravings. Many cravings stem from various sources – lack of sleep, mineral deficiencies, lack of good quality foods or another imbalance. When we eat something sugary, the hormone insulin is secreted by the pancreas to bring blood sugar into cells to be used. However, when that happens, there is a blood sugar spike, which is followed by an energy crash. Eating whole foods and avoiding or limiting white bread, high-fructose corn syrup and other forms of sugar can keep blood sugar balanced.

The amount of protein you require will depend on your goals, how much and how intensely you exercise, your height and body type. A 5'4" woman who does aerobic exercise twice a week will require a much different protein intake than a 6'4" athlete who does strength training. Protein requirements will also change in pregnancy, after surgery and if a person has another preexisting health condition such as kidney disease.

Be patient with yourself and set small goals each week. For

example, maybe one week you can switch from regular soda to kombucha. Another week you could try adding in more fermented foods like kimchi or sauerkraut. Reaching your optimal health is a journey so let's make it a fun one!

Since food addiction is both physiological and psychological, you may also want to use some of the Energy Tools in the Appendix such as Affirmations or Vision Boards. Stress eating is common in many of the clients I see, and I encourage them to do the following:

- **Name that mood** each time you eat. This allows you to identify episodes of emotional eating and see trends. Are you eating out of boredom, frustration, guilt, shame, disappointment?
- **Ride out the storm** of negative emotions. Know that every emotion is temporary. Meditation helps reduce future episodes of impulsively eating out of frustration or stress.
- **Discover healthy coping**. Exercising and talking with a supportive friend. Discover what food gives you. Is it comfort, relief, freedom? Whatever that feeling is that you get from eating, try to find other creative ways to get to that feeling. For example, one of my clients said that being with her friends gave her a sense of freedom and joy. I encouraged her to seek out those opportunities to be with friends, whether that was on the phone or in person.
- **Conquering difficult times is the key to success.** *"This isn't a good time for me to be trying to lose weight."* There will never be a "perfect time" since life is full of chaos. Remove the excuses! You can handle whatever life throws at you!

Applying these concepts will help you gain confidence in being able to break the cycle of food addiction!

Reflection Week 3:

1. Create your own Appetite Scale this week. Decipher when you might need a snack and when you might need a meal. Before you eat anything, jot down the Appetite Scale number you are at and what you are feeling at that time. Ex: Before lunch, 6, ate a snack an hour ago.
2. What are two ways you can decrease cravings for sugar?
3. Practice being aware of what your body needs in three scenarios this week. Write that down in your journal. Ex: I felt a slight headache coming on, had a glass of lemon water and found that I had worked all day without drinking water.

Week 4: Letting Go to Lighten Up!

Overcoming Resistance is the Biggest Hurtle

As a society, we tend to think that we need to fix things physically before any progress begins. I have seen time and time again, that the opposite phenomenon is true. We must look at our mindset, our beliefs and our attitude about something before anything changes.

It seems counterintuitive that I would tell you to "let go" of resistance when it comes to losing weight. Many people think that they need to work really hard, starve themselves and that will lead to success. The opposite is true!

Have you ever tried forcing your child to eat broccoli or a food they hate? They just resist it more! What about having someone, perhaps a nosy family member, push their advice or beliefs onto you? You would resist that too I am sure!

Often, inner resistance to the present moment is what keeps us stuck, frustrated and in a negative mindset. We want to be somewhere else besides work. We would be happier if 20 pounds were gone or we hit the $20 million jackpot! We resist or push against, being present and happy about where we are.

Resistance in physics deals with opposition or friction. For example, electrical resistance is the measure of the degree to which a conductor opposes an electric current through that system. In the military, resistance is the ability of an organized force to stand on the defensive. When you think of internal resistance, you can imagine a tug of war with two people pulling at opposite ends of the rope.

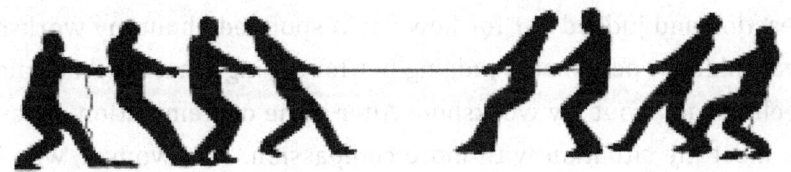

Figure 2. Tug of war

We all have some resistance, and that can fluctuate from day to day. For example, suggestion from an untrusted outside source may cause resistance to new ideas. Imagine a stranger walked up to you on the street and said, *"I think you should start exercising twice a week."* If you wouldn't be completely upset by that, kudos to you! I think most of us would be offended. However, if someone you hire as a health coach were to suggest something similar, your resistance would be much less!

Our internal resistance can prevent us from following through with making healthy choices. Often we resist change, and it can be uncomfortable to start adapting new habits. Are you nodding your head as you read that?

Negative past experiences can create resistance to trying a new approach. I have two examples of this. I was set to conduct a Mindfulness workshop and was at a networking event to share about it. I overheard one of my colleagues mention my workshop to a woman at the networking event. The woman shouted, *"Why would I have someone tell me how to eat mindfully? I already feel terrible about the way I eat! I don't need to feel worse about myself."* My colleague gave me a deer-in-headlights look; she was only trying to help recruit participants for my workshop.

I went home that night feeling many emotions about that woman's reaction and judged her for how she responded about my workshop. I was taking it personally, judging her for saying what she had said and feeling bad about my workshop! After some contemplation, I was able to meet the situation with more compassion. This woman, who I had never met, had so much resistance to the idea of losing weight and getting guidance around eating mindfully. As I replayed the situation in my mind again, I could hear the frustration, pain, disappointment and underlying guilt that this woman had from years and years of failed attempts to regain her health. I let it go, and I felt a lot better. Why? Because I let go of my resistance!

There is so much in between what someone says and what their non-verbal cues say that helps me pick up on what is blocking them. Language is 93% non-verbal. Only 7% is verbal, and the rest comes from gesturing and tonality of a person's voice. In this case, this woman had so much resistance that she was not willing to be open-minded about the workshop.

In another example, I had a client who wanted to make healthy meals for her family but couldn't get moving on making time for planning meals on the weekend. I encouraged her to share more about what her resistance was about. She said, *"Well, I used to love to cook and then over time it just became more of another thing to do."* I could sense the ambivalence she had presently, but could also hear that at one time she did enjoy cooking. I asked her a deliberate question, "What energy are you bringing to cooking? Can you see how you are dreading the experience because of how you feel about it?" A metaphorical light bulb went off. "Yes! I am always stressed and tense, rushing through life and I really do want to slow down and enjoy cooking more."

The more resistance we have, the more we remain stuck because we aren't willing to see things from a new perspective or be flexible. If you tried drilling a hole into a steel plate, you wouldn't get very far because steel is rigid. Your goal is to be malleable and flexible so that you can get "unstuck" and gain momentum in moving toward your goal.

You can tell where your energy is based on how you feel. Ask yourself, *"Does my experience feel easy or difficult?"* Being in "the flow" essentially means being in the zone. Someone in the flow loses track of time, is fully concentrated on what they are doing, and there is a sense of enjoyment attached to it.

Resistance	Flow
Things feel difficult and forced	Things feel easy
Feel tense, contracted, heavy	Feel free, light, expansive
Anxiety, worry and projecting into the future	Presence and enjoyment
Lack of abundance, love, opportunity, success	Presence of abundance, love, opportunity, success
Feeling hard, difficult, forced, upstream, heavy, and complicated.	Feeling easy, light, effortless, downstream, exciting, clear and peaceful.

What would happen if you shifted your energy and perspective around something you have resistance to? In psychology, shifting your perspective is called "cognitive reframing." We all see life through a certain "frame" or lens. Reframing is helpful when you need to change your beliefs about something.

For instance, if I asked you to complete the sentence, "Life is_____, it would be different than your husbands or neighbors. You may fill in the blank as "hard, challenging, a bitch, a crapshoot, unfair" or you may say "exciting, an adventure, thrilling." Depending on your perspective, you would answer that question based on your past experience with life.

Let's say I told you I wanted you to walk on a treadmill for an hour. You may dread that and say, *"I don't like treadmills. I don't have time for that. I hate walking."* What if I told you to watch your favorite movie and walk on the treadmill? Maybe for some of you that wouldn't change a thing. You'd still hate it!

Maybe your shift would be around another variable- talking to a friend, changing the environment and walking outside, plugging in your headphones and listening to an audiobook while you walk. Any of these things can help shift your energy and decrease resistance around doing something that is good for you.

Often we fall subject to *faulty thinking,* and that can sabotage our efforts. Cognitive distortions are another word for this faulty thinking. Distortions are ways that our mind convinces us of something that isn't really true. These inaccurate thoughts are usually used to reinforce negative thinking or emotions — telling ourselves things that sound rational and accurate, but really only serve to keep us feeling bad about ourselves.

Some examples include:

- Black-and-white thinking -
  - o This is also called polarized thinking. We think we have to be perfect or we are a failure; there is no middle ground. Good or bad, black or white, and

either/or categorizations are examples.

- Overgeneralizing -
  - o We come to a conclusion based on a single incident. If something happens once, we expect it to happen over and over again. A person may see a single event as a part of never-ending defeat.
- Negating the positive -
  - o Always focusing on what we've done wrong in a situation instead of what we did good or right.
- Filtering -
  - o Our lens of seeing reality is skewed by a past experience where we experienced pain.
- Jumping to conclusions AKA mind-reading -
  - o We think we can know what people think or feel and why they act the way they do without actually asking.
- Catastrophizing -
  - o Always anticipating negative outcomes is a form of catastrophizing. Exaggerating and expecting disaster to strike is another example. Magnifying or minimizing is yet another way this manifests.
- Personalizing -
  - o A person believes everything others do or say is some kind of direct or personal reaction to them. This also involves comparing ourselves to others.
- "Shoulds" or Judgments -
  - o Having a list of fixed or rigid rules about how others should behave or how we should behave. People who break the rules make us angry, and we feel guilty when we violate the rules.
  - o Example, "I shouldn't eat that. I should exercise." The emotional consequence is guilt. When a person directs *should statements* at others, they feel anger,

frustration, and resentment.

- Blaming -
  - o Holding others responsible for our pain OR blaming ourselves for every problem. No one can "make us" feel a certain way. We have complete control of our emotions.
- Heaven's Reward Fallacy -
  - o Expecting sacrifice and self-denial to pay off as if someone is keeping score; we then feel bitter when the reward doesn't come.

If you are stressed, creative solutions often seem unavailable. Opening up your perspective, or in other words, decreasing your resistance, will open up so many options for you. You will no longer need to feel stressed, tense or ambivalent about making good choices for yourself. You will begin to be more aware of how you feel moment to moment.

Start to notice your own inner resistance to life in general. If things seem very difficult, or you need to work hard or struggle, you'll know you are in a resistant, fearful energy. On the other hand, if things seem easy and have a flow to it, you'll know you are in the flow, aligned with positive energy that will get you to your goal!

The Power of Surrender

When I first came across the research of Dr. David Hawkins, it completely changed the way I saw disease and healing. Little did I realize that he had a whole series of books, notably one called *Letting Go: The Pathway of Surrender.*

The main theme in *Letting Go* is that when we hold onto negative emotions like shame, guilt, fear, grief, apathy and so on, we suffer. When we can begin to let go of judging our feelings and be the silent witness, we literally lighten up.

I have seen these patterns in each one of my clients and in myself. Hawkins refers to these emotions as being tied to each other, not a singular, stand-alone emotion. For example, anger and guilt normally wire together. We feel angry and silently judge others and ourselves and subconsciously feel guilty about it. Letting go of these emotions, one by one, will help us restore our energy and vitality.

Think about how you feel when you judge someone or participate in gossip. I am assuming that you feel drained, guilty because you know it is not positive and maybe even a sense of shame. Setting boundaries and refusing to participate in negative talk to yourself and to others will help you feel lighter.

Originally, Sigmund Freud used the word *ego* to mean a sense of self but later revised it to mean a set of psychic functions such as judgment, tolerance, control, planning, defense, synthesis of information, intellectual functioning, and memory. The ego is not your amigo and *edges God out*! Your Higher Self is your infinitely wise self that can access spiritual truths and lead you to your best life. The ego part of you seeks to compete, drag you down and keep you small and stuck. Your Higher Self seeks to encourage you and help you onto the next part of your journey.

Some characteristics of the ego and the Higher Self:

The "ego"	"Higher Self"
Manipulates, controls, forces	Allows, surrenders, true power
Never satisfied	Content with what is
Comes from fear	Comes from love

Looks at the material, external	Looks at spiritual, internal
Critical, "tough love"	Encouraging, supportive
Problem focused	Solution focused

Of course, most people are not aware of these systems operating within them.

There are many ways in which the human mind creates issues through the ego:

- Needing to be right and make others wrong
- Needing approval
- Gossiping
- Complaining
- Being a victim
- Being a martyr
- Having to be superior to others
- Needing to look good and avoid looking bad
- Defending your position

The list goes on. When we have these patterns and emotions running, it is important to simply notice and surrender to them instead of holding on and feeling guilty that we have them. Don't make it mean anything; simply notice these human reactions. Each interaction you experience impacts your energy. For example, if someone cuts you off in traffic you may have some choice words with them. You may then repeat the story to your coworkers, spouse and others multiple times during the day, giving the story more energy and power. Instead, you can choose to let go and realize that you are preserving your energy and staying in your power.

The word *"surrender"* is synonymous with letting go and you may have various associations with it. Perhaps to you, it means giving up, backing down, caving in, etc. However, in this context, it will mean you are releasing and allowing energy to move. Hanging on and resisting feelings will cause them to stay stuck in your body. What we resist, persists. If we think, *"I shouldn't be feeling this way,"* it means that our emotions are not welcome. Instead, we can let them go and be a nonjudgmental witness to them.

This is the major goal of meditation. We can allow our feelings to come up to the surface and let them go. One of my early therapists likened this practice to watching clouds pass by on a summer day. We can be a witness to the clouds (feelings) passing by and we do not have to react to it.

I encourage many of my clients to discover where they feel stressed energy in their body. Does it go to your shoulders? Your heart? Your stomach? Becoming more aware of where your body holds this energy will allow you to breathe into it and *let it go.*

As you go throughout your week, keep note of the ways in which you need to be right and make others wrong. Be mindful of your inner resistance and actively choose to release the energy. As you become more aware, you will find a deep sense of peace in letting things go. You will find that you want inner peace rather than being right or defending yourself.

Reflection Week 4:

1. What do you notice you have or have had resistance to?
2. What are your beliefs about being healthy?
3. Highlight the cognitive distortions you most commonly fall prey to. Describe two situations where you have distorted reality in that scenario.
4. What are two ways you can let go more this week?

5. What are the differences between the ego self and your Higher self?

Week 5: Finding Stillness in an Over-Stimulated World

Calming the Stress Response

I used to live in Brooklyn in a six-story apartment building across from a busy subway station. I avoided getting on the subway from 8-9AM and 5-6PM. You can probably guess why. Everyone was in a rush, and people literally squeezed into the subway cars like sardines, sometimes even pushing people out of the way to get in. That good ol' NYC subway... It caused me a lot of anxiety.

I also had to get up every morning to move my car for street cleaning at 7:30AM. If you were a minute late to your car, there would be a huge orange parking ticket to say good morning. There was so much noise in my building, as I was right by the lobby and heard every sound reverberating through the hallways. Needless to say, living in Brooklyn was extremely stressful for me, but at the time it all seemed normal!

I didn't realize how much my environment had been stressing me out until I moved to a quiet suburb in Western PA. Can you relate to this where you live? Perhaps your work environment is a stressful. There is so much going on in this world, and you can easily find out by turning on the news, reading a newspaper or listening to the radio.

Also, you may have other responsibilities like kids to take care of, jobs to do, and other tasks, errands and projects to complete. Oh yea, and you are supposed to make time to keep yourself healthy. It has been estimated that 90% of all doctor visits are due to stress. With the advancement of technology and the use of Smartphones, the stress response is heightened even more. Various studies have shown that there is a direct correlation between social media use and anxiety levels.

When our bodies get stressed, many hormones like adrenaline, cortisol, and norepinephrine are released as a result. Cortisol is a hormone that is released from the adrenal glands located on top of each kidney. Cortisol is responsible for rapid aging, anxiety, weight gain, and deplete your energy levels among other impacts. Yikes! Let's lower cortisol.

In order for your body to return to "homeostasis" or normal levels of function, you need to address stress. Yes, that rhymes! Stress can seem to come from many sources such as family or work conflict, financial worry, interpersonal relationship stress and I've even seen the holidays as a top source of stress! The holiday season is a time when we remember loved ones who have passed and try to get shopping, wrapping, cleaning and cooking done. I get it!

Stress and inflammation go hand in hand. From the Latin, "*inflammare*", inflammation means heat, swelling or redness or literally "to set on fire." Imagine having to create a fire with only twigs. Constant rubbing and friction creates fire.

The same concept can be applied to our body. Constant stress leads to friction and chronic inflammation, which can have detrimental health effects on the body. There are two opposing systems in the body to control our stress response - the "fight or "flight" or sympathetic nervous system and the "rest and digest" or parasympathetic nervous system. Those are just two fancy terms for the gas pedal and the brake pedal of our body.

When we are stressed, the gas pedal, or sympathetic nervous system, is activated. We experience sweaty palms, increased heart rate, and reduced blood flow to our digestive tract. On the other hand, the brake pedal, or parasympathetic nervous system, helps us "rest and digest." Most Americans are so stressed that they don't even digest their food.

Many of my clients feel that they have so many things to do and very little time for themselves. When we look at their schedule, there tend to be a few ways they are sabotaging their time, and often we find optimal ways to make use of that time.

For example, I had a client who used to get up at 5AM every day and look at her finances. She would spend about 10 minutes moseying around the house, cleaning up from the day prior and then 20 minutes looking at financial statements. She quickly realized that this 30-minute time frame could be better spent. Did looking at the finances every day truly serve her? She decided to get laser-focused on her goal to lose weight and look at the finances once a week. Instead, she dedicated her mornings to either prayer/meditation and reading or exercising on the treadmill for 30 minutes.

Often when we feel stressed, there are limited options, and we feel "stuck." There are things we can change, however! Just like my client, you can look at your schedule and map out how you spend your day. Not every minute has to have a productive activity. For example, you can map out your relaxation time too! Having your entire schedule physically in front of you also eliminates any excuses of "I don't have time."

We tend to think that stress is due to external forces. However, the way we perceive circumstances is within our control, and thus we can choose to be stressed or not. After continuous "stress" our internal state is always on guard looking for the next metaphorical shoe to drop. Our response to stress depends on our proneness to it.

Picture a dial that goes from 1 to 10, 1 being absolutely no stress or internal pressure and 10 being extreme stress and internal pressure. Each one of us has a different level of internal pressure from past experiences and unresolved emotions. If you are at an 8 and something in your external environment stresses you out, you will *perceive* it to be extremely stressful. If you are normally at a 2, that person may perceive that same scenario as not stressful at all.

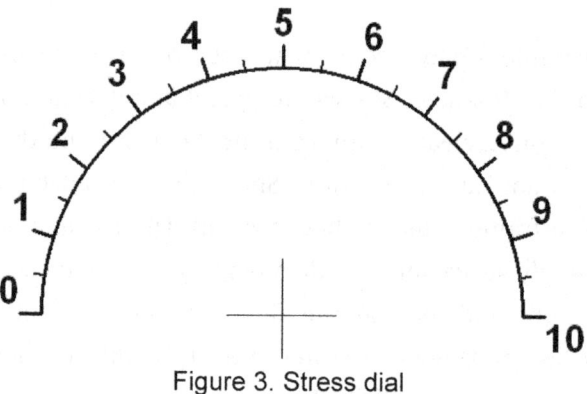

Figure 3. Stress dial

Imagine a kettle full of boiling hot water. When the pressure gets to be too much, it is at full capacity, and the steam starts coming through the tiny hole in the kettle. That is how most people live who calibrate at higher levels of baseline stress. There is already so much internal pressure that, from their perspective, they *feel* stressed.

Witnessing your emotions through a practice like meditation and progressively letting go of those negative feelings can help you reduce that "internal pressure." When you can let go of some of that pressure, you lower your vulnerability to external stressors. You'll notice things that used to bother you don't anymore. You will notice a sense of calm pervading your life.

There are many ways to dial down stress and recharge your metaphorical batteries. One method is utilizing halotherapy or salt therapy. Halotherapy was accidently discovered after cave workers in Poland were seen to have less incidence of respiratory illness. There are many salt caves around the U.S. that are meant to provide a relaxing haven for people seeking to relieve stress and improve their health. These salt caves mimic the microclimate of natural salt caves.

What's the big deal about a salt cave?

Negative ions from salt act to reduce inflammation, combat free radical damage and promote healing. Negative ions are oxygen molecules with an added electron. They are odorless, tasteless, and invisible molecules that we inhale in abundance in certain environments such as near waterfalls, at the beach and in a salt cave. High concentrations of negative ions are essential for high energy and positive mood.

You have experienced the relaxing effect of negative ions while being at a beach. Being in a salt cave for 45 minutes is equivalent to the exposure you would get with 3 days at the beach!!

The benefits aren't just theoretical. A study in the May 2017 issue of *Pediatric Pulmonology* found that children with mild asthma who went for two halotherapy sessions per week for seven weeks gained greater improvements in their asthma symptoms than a control group did. Also, a small study in a 2014 issue of the *Journal of Medicine and Life* found that when patients with chronic bronchial conditions underwent halotherapy, it triggered anti-inflammatory mechanisms and stimulation of phagocytosis, a process in which cells called phagocytes engulf bacterial or viral particles to destroy them.

Halotherapy can help:

- Skin conditions

- Respiratory health
- Reduce inflammation
- Boost immunity
- Reduce stress and boost mood

Visit bitly.com/saltcaveresource to find a salt cave near you. Always check with your medical provider or a qualified healthcare professional prior to trying any new regimen or treatment.

The Mind Body Connection

When I began reading David Hawkin's Power Vs. Force, it truly changed the way I saw disease. Hawkins proved that our emotional state calibrates at a certain frequency and since we are energetic beings, that frequency could easily be measured.

All living creatures generate and emit energy. Photons of light, electromagnetic frequencies, heat, and sound are all emitted from our bodies in direct relationship to our internal states. This remarkable, subtle system of exchange contains a wealth of information.

Kirlian photography, for example, shows the energy field around a certain object. Kirlian photographic analysis combines high voltage, high frequency, ultra low current, electrical fields and photographic techniques to make visible subtle energy fields interacting with living and non-living objects of study. Our internal states impact our physical body.

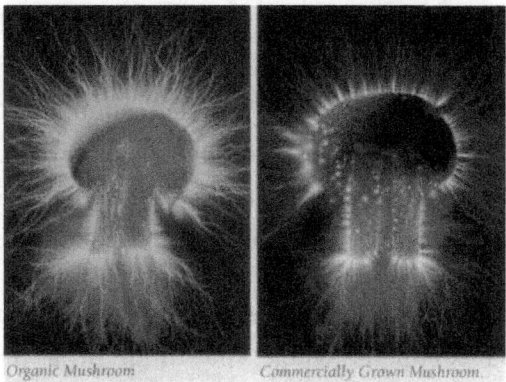

Organic Mushroom   *Commercially Grown Mushroom*

Figure 4. Kirlian Photography

As you can see in the diagram above, the organic mushroom has more energy around it, indicating that it has a higher energetic frequency. Chiropractic philosophy teaches that correction of vertebral subluxation reduces nerve interference and promotes health. It has been further taught that the chiropractic adjustment liberates life force when such subluxation is reduced, thereby allowing the body's own self-regulatory mechanisms to achieve normality.

Even our thoughts are energy. All of our thoughts, beliefs and past experiences form the subconscious mind. About 90% of our consciousness is subconscious and therefore hidden from view. This explains why we may want to achieve certain things in life, but we self-sabotage or are held back and don't know why.

Hypnosis is a powerful technique that can help a person align their subconscious beliefs with what they desire. Think of the conscious and subconscious as playing tug-of-war. Five to 10% of the force is on the conscious side, and 90-95% is on the subconscious side pulling you back to old beliefs, behaviors, and patterns. Other tools like Emotional Freedom Technique (EFT) can work with the subconscious to release trapped emotions.

Since everything is energy, including our thoughts, we draw into our lives what we predominantly think about. The brain scans your environment to confirm your underlying, subconscious beliefs. For example, if you are constantly worried about "not having enough money," you will attract those circumstances into your life until you change the underlying belief structure. Hypnosis or EFT can help you reprogram your subconscious to attract more money in this case.

If you need proof that your thoughts impact your physical body, think of what happens when you think of a delicious piece of cheesecake. Does your mouth start to salivate? What happens when your boss calls you into his or her office? Doesn't your heart start to beat? This is a direct example of how your thoughts control your body!

Your words and beliefs are powerful and create your reality. If you continue to say, "I have X disease" or "I am fat" that will perpetuate the problem. As you change your language and inner feelings about yourself, your external environment will change. This is opposite to what most people think. They think, "I need to lose 50 pounds and *then* I will be happy." "I'll be happy when I finally get that raise."

The laws of the universe don't work that way! Author and speaker Esther Hicks teaches about the law of attraction and getting into a good feeling place or the "vortex." The vortex is aligning yourself with source energy, God or what you choose to call that energy. When you are in the vortex you feel aligned with joy, inspiration, and passion. The more negative emotion we feel, the further away we are from the vortex. This ties into the chapter on resistance. As you *allow*, *let go* and *surrender* you align with that vortex.

As mentioned, there are ways to get your subconscious mind on board to align your desires with your conscious mind. There are other techniques listed in **Appendix C** of this book such as meditation, vision boarding, affirmations and so on. However, we are focusing on how to get you to a good feeling place in a different way.

Imagine you think of your pet or a pet you've had before. How do you feel about this pet? When I think of my long-haired dachshund Penny, I smile instantly. Why is that? Why do we smile at babies and dogs? There are no resistant thoughts there like guilt, resentment, blame or envy. Finding something to appreciate will expand your good feelings. Over time, you have developed many opinions and attitudes, and beliefs about yourself, that when activated, hold you outside the vortex. It is easier to get inside the vortex by focusing upon other subjects that are easier for you to feel good about.

Another way to get into the vortex is to focus upon that which you want, not what you don't want. If you say, "*I don't want to get fat*" the brain just hears "want fat." Affirm what you want and be clear about it. By understanding that your everyday emotions impact your life, you will become more deliberate in how you live your life. Create a powerful declaration!

Practicing gratitude, praying, meditating and appreciating something will pull you into that good feeling place.

The reason why most of my clients have stayed stuck with other "diet programs" is because they have tried changing everything from the outside instead of from the inside. Only focusing on shakes, skinny wraps, topical solutions simply provides a temporary fix.

Your mind affects your body. Period. Gain control of your thoughts, and you will see your physical reality alter in a way you've never imagined. Do this for any area in your life – relationships, health, career, family. When you change your thoughts around something, you will see the circumstances gradually change and shift.

Silencing the Inner Critic

One of the most prevalent beliefs I hear clients say is that they doubt themselves. This doubt spans across many aspects of their life, not just in food choices. They may have trouble deciding on important decisions, setting boundaries and knowing what they want.

At the core of self-doubt is lack of trust in oneself. Often this lack of self-trust can stem from various circumstances that happen throughout life that cause us to doubt ourselves. For example, maybe you trusted your heart when you had a crush on someone in college, and they broke your heart. Or maybe you thought you landed a great job opportunity only to find out that it wasn't exactly what you wanted.

We make meaning out of our past experiences. You may say, "I'm big boned" or "I've always been heavy" or "Obesity runs in my family." That doesn't mean anything! Holding onto those limiting beliefs prevents you from being fully engaged in the process of getting healthy. You think, "What's the point? I've been heavy all of my life." This is a disempowering mindset and perpetuates future failures.

Completing the past is necessary to move forward with a clean slate. Forgiving yourself for anything you did or did not do is a great exercise to complete the past. Allow yourself to see all of the faulty belief systems that are running in your mind. Let them go!

After you've completed the past, you can move forward in a powerful way with a fresh perspective on self-trust. In order to strengthen the muscle of trusting yourself, you need to be able to know your true inner guidance and listen to it. The challenge is that many of us are constantly bombarded with distractions.

We live in a world full of noise driven by car horns, traffic, emails, texts and social media. With so much noise and activity, our bodies become over-stimulated and do not function optimally. Anxiety and depression are more common with social media use, and researchers have found that the longer you spend on social media, the more likely you are to be depressed.

We hear many voices throughout the day – bosses, spouses, friends, family, people on the news and more. Everyone has opinions about what we *should* and *shouldn't do.* We get this messaging from magazines, on t.v. and from our peer groups. It can be challenging to hear *our own true inner voice* when there is so much stimulation occurring.

How can we hear the voice of our inner selves?

Many of us have competing voices inside of us that usually begin with the words, "What if?" Whenever you ask a "What if?" question, let that be your indicator that you are operating from fear. On one hand, we want to be healthier, succeed in our career and be in loving relationships. On the other hand, there can be old belief structures that tell us distorted messages. Silencing competing voices is key to being able to hear and trust your inner voice.

Some competing messages might be:

- You aren't enough
- Not enough money in the bank, not enough friends on Facebook, not enough nice clothes, big house or other material things.
- Bringing up how you've "failed in the past"
- Believing you are not safe and things happen to you
- What if I lose my job?
- What if my husband leaves me?
- What if I can never reach my health goal?

All of these competing messages are lies that come from fear. Being able to discern these voices will help you redirect your focus back to the truth, which is that you are enough, you are supported and guided, and you are safe. Think about this: What if I showed you a picture of a $100 bill and asked you if it was fake or real? Since it is simply a picture, there would be no way of telling whether or not it was fake or real. Bank tellers know when a bill is fake not because they've studied fakes, but because they have studied the real thing.

The same concept can be applied to hearing your inner voice. Get to know yourself. Get to know God and your Higher Self and develop a relationship with Him. Surround yourself with positive friends who can support you in this endeavor. Who you surround yourself with is imperative! It's been said that we are the sum of the 5 people we spend the most time with.

We impact each other with the words we say, the energy we bring to conversations and the actions we take. If you are honest with yourself, are you surrounding yourself with people who complain, gossip and are negative? Are *you* one of those people? Or are you around people who are constantly improving and are positive? The choice is yours! Be careful not to place judgment on yourself or others as you are just becoming aware of this next layer of "releasing" negativity.

You may have been friends with people for years! Yet if you continue to allow negativity in your life, it will drain you.

Developing healthy boundaries helps you preserve your energy and improve your health. Think of all of the things you can do when you set good boundaries! You can start to work on that book you've been wanting to write or learn guitar like you've always wanted to. When you set boundaries, you have more time to focus on your life purpose and doing things that bring *you* joy.

When we do not have healthy boundaries, it is easy for people to take advantage of us and treat us poorly. Boundaries are a form of self-respect and show people where the line is that they cannot cross. Each of us will have our own map of what that looks like to be clear about our boundaries.

Realize that it is okay to say "No" to certain things. Picture a waiter who has to clean up a table. He can balance 3 or 4 plates at the most. After adding on the 5th plate, he drops them all. This is what I mean by saying 'No.' If you are constantly stressed and putting your energy in 5 different places, you will feel overwhelmed, and this can trigger feeling out of control. You aren't a failure because you "can't handle it." You are actually more effective if you balance 3 or 4 plates well.

As you create boundaries, people in your life may push back. They are so used to you saying, "Yes" that when they hear "No" it may be an adjustment. A natural feeling that might show up is guilt because perhaps you haven't taken this step before. Know that it will subside as you build the muscle of boundary setting. If you find that certain people aren't respecting your boundaries, you have several options.

You can set healthy boundaries by limiting time with that person or group. Setting healthy boundaries means you honor and take care of yourself and protect your energy. If you talk to a friend on the phone who complains about an hour and barely lets you get a word in, limit the conversation. Let them know upfront that you only have a certain amount of time to talk.

1. You can distance yourself from that person and back off from spending time with them. When you do this, they may not be aware on the conscious level what is happening. Some relationships simply fall apart on their own. Some get stronger.
2. You can have an honest conversation around what has not been working in the relationship. In order to stay in your power, don't go into it blaming or saying how they are wrong.

You are owning your feelings and naming the behavior. For example, you could say *"I feel disconnected from you when you cut me off while I am talking. I want us to be able to hear each other clearly."* You want to make sure you aren't saying, *"I hate when you cut me off!"* That will immediately put the person on the defensive.

This week, notice where you need to set healthy boundaries, whether with yourself or others in your life. Get excited; you just finished another week!

Reflection Week 5:

1. How can you create more stillness in your life this week?
2. Track your stress level each day this week. Do you notice any patterns of periods where you feel more stressed?
3. What are some ways to reclaim your power and dial down your internal stress?
4. Write out the major areas of your life. Relationships, Career, Family, Friends, Self, etc. Be honest and see where you may be giving too much of yourself in one area. If we are not balanced, it will cost you in another area, such as health.

Week 6: Stopping the Cycle of Pain

Asking Empowering Questions

I stepped up to the microphone on the wooden stage and cleared my throat. Seventy-five pair of eyes remained fixated on me as I shifted my weight from right to left. Throat clearing. Heart pumping. Voice quivering. *"So...I find myself dating the same people over and over again. They are all unavailable. I have an eating disorder where I wake up every night and binge eat."* Complete silence filled the room. Could they hear my heart beating over the microphone?

"What do you feel guilty about? It's clear your life isn't workable," said the man with the squinty eyes and big teeth asked from the center of the room.

"Well...I left my dad's pharmacy, and he kicked me out of the house when I was 23," I said, starting to get choked up.

"And you feel that he shouldn't have done that, right?"

"Yes. It eats at me."

"Well good. You were 23. Time to grow up," he answered. Gulp.

He continued. *"You need to stop blaming your parents. You are 26 years old, Christina. Have you forgiven them?"*

"Yes."

"Have you forgiven yourself?"

"No."

"You are punishing yourself for betraying them. Dating bad boys, having an eating disorder. The way to get back at them is not to have your life work. Am I right?"

"Yes..." I said, almost reflexively.

"So here is what you are going to do. You are going to call your parents and tell them you love them. You are also going to tell them they don't need to worry about you anymore."

Awakening is defined as an act or moment of becoming suddenly aware of something. That day at the Landmark Forum in New York City, *I woke up.* Sometimes we are too close to ourselves to see things clearly. The definition of insanity is doing the same thing over again and expecting a different result. Yet, most of us continue to perpetuate these situations.

At that point in my life, I was stuck dating unavailable men that abused me emotionally and put me down. I had no idea why I was attracting that type of person into my life. A friend had recommended Landmark Education, and I had resisted for some time. When I finally mustered up the courage to go, I wished I had done it sooner!

That day in 2014 my life changed because I took my power back. I saw how I had blamed my parents for many events that had occurred in my childhood and in doing so, I gave my power away. Don't parents always get blamed? I noticed that I had not forgiven myself for the incident that had happened in 2012. The guilt, shame, and fear inside of me attracted low-quality individuals and circumstances into my life.

The minute I forgave myself and took my power back, my life changed.

After that several things changed for me.

1. I began healing my eating disorder and treating my body with respect. I found a balance in eating, neither depriving nor binging on food. I exercised because it helped me feel good, not to punish myself.
2. I grew to have a better relationship with my parents because nothing else was in the way.
3. I stepped up in my business and published my first book, *Revealing Your Inner Radiance: Healing through the Heart.* I traveled to Bali that year with a Writer's Retreat to do so.

Holding onto resentment is like drinking poison and hoping the other person dies. Resentment has a cost. It costs you love and affinity for others, your health and precious time. Don't let old grudges, resentment or "stories" get in the way of closeness with family or friends. ***Remember, even if it doesn't seem like it, it costs you in your health and happiness!!***

Most of us walk through life with stories about traffic, our family, friends and how life "should be." We repeat patterns over and over again without understanding why. The world continues to send us lessons through people so that we can wake up to our power, freedom, and self-expression.

Often we are not aware of what is holding us in the pattern because it is a "blind spot" and we can't see it. In my case, I was repeating a cycle I was familiar with – feeling guilty and punishing myself. In the vicious cycle, we are on a hamster wheel without knowing how to break free. We attach meaning to things that have occurred in the past and literally create our lives. When we relive the past throughout pain cycle, our lives don't work.

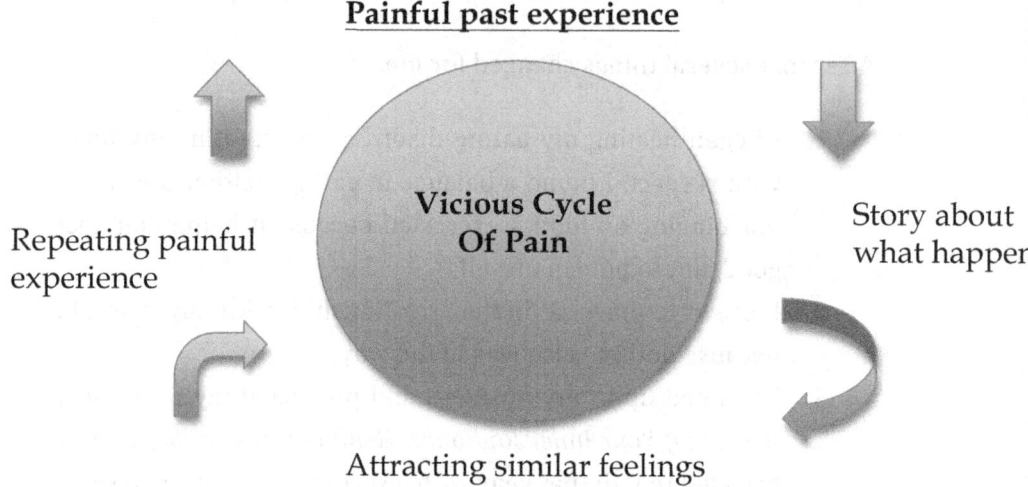

Painful past experience

Vicious Cycle
Of Pain

Repeating painful
experience

Story about
what happen

Attracting similar feelings
and circumstances

Your life cannot work when you are punishing others or yourself from past experiences. When you do this, you give your power away to the past and to those who hurt you or if you have hurt others. To reclaim your power, you need to take ownership of your life and stop blaming others. We are all doing our best in each moment and operate at different levels of awareness. Once you have an awakening, you will never be the same. Your life will begin to work because you actually have authentic power.

How to discover and stop your pain cycle:

1. What is the area of your life that is not currently workable? Ex: Relationships, career, health.
2. What is your "story" about that area of your life. Ex: Men can't be trusted. I can never lose weight because of my metabolism. I'm too old now.
3. What was something that happened in the past that lead you to develop that story? The first thing that pops in your mind is usually the source of the painful experience.

4. How does this cycle replay in your current life? *If you cannot discover this for yourself, I can help in your next coaching session.

5. How can you forgive yourself or others for incidents that have happened in the past? Take an inventory of who you have not forgiven and make an action plan to have meaningful conversations with them. Put the past in the past! You will notice a lightness in your body after you do this, I promise!

Sometimes you may not be able to see your pain cycle or what is holding you back in general. Why is that? There are three levels of knowing I'd like to highlight for you.

1. **We know what we know.** I know how to ride a bike, drive a car and brush my teeth.

2. **We know what we don't know.** I don't know how to perform brain surgery, and I certainly don't know how to fly a plane.

3. **We don't know what we don't know.** This is where it get's interesting. This is also known as our "blindspot."

Three Levels of Knowing

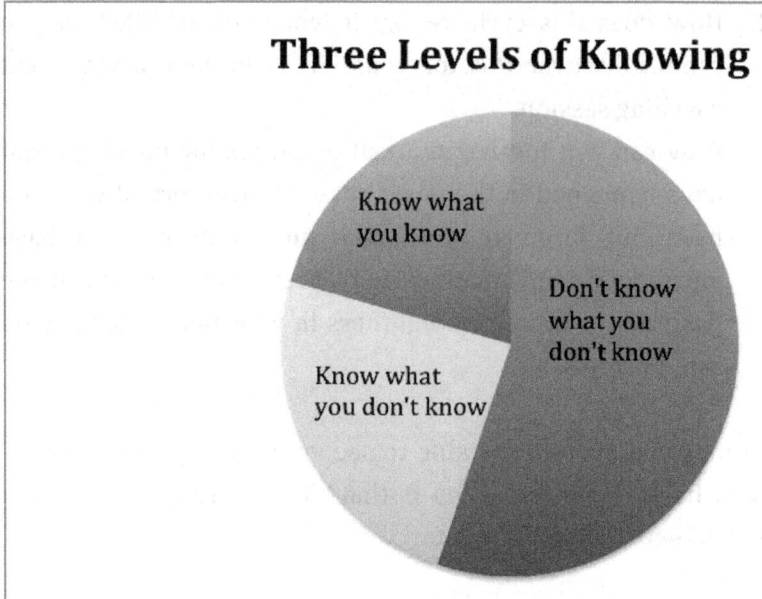

Figure 5. Levels of Knowing

The majority of what we don't know we don't know is otherwise known as a "blindspot." Think of the blindspot when you drive a car. You can't always see the blindspot unless you actually turn your head and look. Your blindspot is hidden from your view, and thus, you cannot always see what is blocking you.

Coaching is so powerful because we don't know what we don't know and the coach can see the blindspot. Other people may be able to see the problem or block when you can't. Certain habits or language patterns may be holding you back. As you saw in the Resistance chapter, the way you speak can empower you or disarm you to get to your goal.

Having an accountability partner and coach helps you tremendously in this area. If you are my coaching client, you have already seen the power of how coaching helps you see what you can't see for yourself.

It can be scary to look at ourselves and see how we sabotage our efforts or what habits we have become accustomed to. However, having a compassionate, curious approach is the way to go. So many of us have berated ourselves for years with negative self-talk, stories of not being good enough and so on.

When you embark on any personal growth journey, it requires courage, consistency, and honesty. It is easy to listen to that inner critic that tells you:

"Look, you are failing again. Why do I always do this?"

"What's the point of trying?"

"I've done it before, and it's never worked out for me."

Do any of those beliefs sound familiar? Instead of asking *disempowering* questions to yourself, rephrase it. Start by asking *empowering* questions that will help you get to your goal.

Your **BELIEFS** →create your **EMOTIONS**→ create your **RESULTS**.

What would happen if you started loving and approving of yourself? What would it take for you to heal some of those beliefs from the past? What if you could let go of the image you hold in your mind about yourself and your limitations? What if you started noticing what you do *right* instead of looking at what you did *wrong?*

As you begin to be more kind to yourself, you will notice good things coming into your life. Like attracts like! Don't be surprised if you start receiving more compliments, praise or abundance in your life after or during your reading this book. You are on a journey of taking the best care of yourself! Jot down all of the good things that you receive.

What's the Big Deal About Judgments?

This entire book is about increasing your awareness of what you hold onto and releasing it to get out of your own way. Another habit that can get in the way of achieving your goals is judging yourself and others.

Energy healer and coach, Christie Marie Sheldon often speaks about how judgments impact our energy. What blocks us from getting what we want most is our self-judgment and judgment of how things "should be." When you set an intention, everything that has been getting in your way will bubble up to the surface to be healed and released.

I often see this come up in my weight loss clients. They will be excited in the beginning of their journey, but somewhere in the 3rd or 4th week, they hit a roadblock. Maybe they go on vacation and "fall off the wagon" or they find themselves getting too enmeshed in work and make excuses for not following through on goals. They immediately place judgment on themselves and beat themselves up for not doing it perfectly or saying, "I should have done XYZ."

Dr. Hawkins scale of consciousness has levels that fall into two categories: expanded or contracted. Judgment is a contracted state and will not lead to solutions that work. Whenever you feel yourself judging, you will often feel negative and heavy because you are in a contracted energy state. You will know your judgments when you hear yourself saying the words "should" or "ought to." Another key phrase might be "I can't do that."

When you judge yourself, you are operating from fear instead of love. When you judge others, you are also judging yourself because we are all connected. Even small judgments of your coworkers, family or friends lower your energy state.

Imagine you start each day with $1000 in your energy bank. Each time you judge someone, you are taking money away from yourself. Maybe you silently criticize your boss each time you see him or her. Choosing to do this depletes your energy bank account and winds up leaving you disempowered, frustrated and sad.

When you catch yourself saying these phrases, ask yourself, "Is that really true?" Are you judging things out of your life?

Notice how you feel when you drop these judgments about yourself and instead invite in compassion, acceptance, and love. Stopping gossip, complaining and negative talk will leave room for good things to enter your life. As you begin shifting your perception of yourself and the world around you, you will feel lighter and free.

Also, pay attention to the words you use. I decided to stop cursing after having a serious conversation with my Landmark leader. I'm not a sailor, but it had become habitual, and internally I knew I wanted to change that habit.

"Honey, when you curse, you lower your energy. When you stop, you will see how many good things are attracted to you. I promise!" said my Landmark leader.

Intuitively I had known that my mouth could get the best of me and it did lower my frequency. Yet, somehow the habit stuck and I had kept the pattern going. After that conversation, I vowed to "test it out" and stopped cursing immediately. No 'I'm trying.' I just stopped.

Within a few days, I knew she was right. I had dropped my judgments and eliminated cursing or negative talk from my vocabulary. Whenever someone started complaining or gossiping, I changed the subject. I enrolled my family into this "no cursing" plan and saw incredible results in my business and in my relationships.

Make the decision to stop all negative talk to yourself and others. When you catch yourself going back to your old ways, stop yourself! Not only will you start attracting positive experiences, but your health will also improve. The week after I stopped cursing, I kept hearing from friends and family "Wow – you are glowing, Christina!" You lighten up when you let go of negative talk.

Reflection Week 6:

1. List your judgments. Make a list of your judgments on an index card or in your phone for 1 week. Notice if there are patterns in what your judgments are.
2. Add gratitude. Reframe your thoughts and focus on appreciation and gratitude for that person or that item.
3. Ask yourself, "What would it take to _____?" Reclaim my health, be open to love, start my new book, etc. When you ask an open-ended question, your brain can come up with creative solutions.
4. Where are your "should" statements? Where are you making excuses that you don't have enough time/money/energy to complete something?

Week 7: Raising Your Frequency

Raising Your Vibration: The Secret to Lighten Up

Everything is energy. If I were to hook you up to an EKG, you would be able to see the waves of your heart's energy on a monitor. This is a vibrational universe comprised of atoms and other fancy physics terms. We are energy, or light beings, and can even tune into each other to tell what is going on internally. You can walk into a room and feel if your husband or wife is upset. When you do this, you are picking up on his/her energy!

Why do I bring up talk about energy? Is this a fluffy, woo woo book? No! According to many studies, your attitude and frequent emotional patterns can have a huge impact on your health and well-being. For example, heart disease has been linked to Type A personality traits such as stress, anger and holding onto resentment.

Do you remember the Scale of Consciousness at the beginning of the book? Anything above the level of 200 (Courage) calibrates with self-promoting behaviors, while anything below lead to self-destructive behaviors.

The higher your vibration, the happier you are, the more "light" you feel and the stronger connection you have with your true self. A tiny dose of physics here...When particles are dense and heavy, they vibrate slowly. However, when particles are light, they vibrate at a faster rate. You can tell something is true based on how light or heavy the statement feels in your body. Your energy will feel heavy if you are not in alignment with the truth and mostly operating from the ego. This is HUGE and one of the biggest reasons why I wrote this book.

Imagine your check engine light goes off. You might bring your car to a mechanic and see what is going on. Now, the mechanic would not look on the outside of the car for the problem. He would look on the inside to see if the oil needed to be changed or something else was wrong. You can liken that example to your body! Imagine if all of this time you have been trying to fix an internal problem by manipulating things externally. It hasn't worked!

Aligning with your highest self and releasing distorted belief systems, fear, negativity, anger, resentment, judgment, shame and so on will lead you to optimal health. It will literally lighten you up and also inspire many others around you. That is the definition of enlightenment if you break down the word. En-lighten-ment means embodying more light!

We are much more than just our physical body. We are energetic, spiritual beings living in a physical body. As you begin to look at each layer of your body – physical, mental, emotional and spiritual- you will unravel and heal your distorted belief systems. Raising your vibration is imperative to dissolve old beliefs, heal and integrate your true self. There are many tools to help you raise your frequency!

Here are some examples to "lighten up!"

1. **Use Gratitude.**
   - Say, "I am so grateful and thankful that this is in my life."
   - This does not mean you are unaware of the fears or

realities of life, but you FOCUS on what you do have.

- Keep a gratitude journal where you write down the 5 things you are grateful for each day. See Gratitude exercise in Appendix.

2. **Eat high-vibrational foods**.

- Use the 80/20 rule—where 80% of what you eat has a high nutrient density, and 20% of what you consume can be a treat.
- Review High Vibrational Food List from **Week 2**

3. **Play more and laugh!**

- Color with your nephew, blow bubbles, go on a trampoline—make a list of the things that you loved doing as a child and DO THEM!
- Laughter is the best medicine! Do more of it! Whether you watch comedians, laugh with friends or play with your puppy, laughter is healing.
- Many adults have the limiting belief that we need to be stern, serious and "practical." This is far from the truth. Keeping a youthful glow and spirit means connecting with your inner child and having fun!

4. **Clear and delete any negative thought** that comes into your mind

- Notice your ego mind telling you things and realize that these fears are not true! Fears stand for Forget Everything And Run—anything below 200 on the Energy Vibration Scale is life depleting. Insert a positive thought!

5. **Open your heart.** The heart energy center (chakra) is the conduit to allow all other energies to flow.

- The heart is at the center of the entire body and is the channel for the lower 3 chakras (physical chakras) and the higher 3 chakras (spiritual chakras). Allowing your heart to open through essential oils (Joy, Rose oil), forgiveness, compassion, and generosity will allow your heart to heal.

- When your heart opens, you begin quickly manifesting love, abundance, and peace in your life.

6. **Meditate for 10 minutes a day.**

- Since most of the time, our minds are bouncing around from thought to thought, quieting the mind raises your vibration.

7. **Examine your limiting beliefs with a coach, mentor or therapist.**

- This is my passion! I want to see people happy, healthy and thriving. We may think that we can "do it alone," but this is not true! We see the world through a certain lens that shapes our reality. Having a coach that can help you compassionately and objectively move through the "blocks" in your life.

- Examine what areas in your life you feel "stuck"— health/wellness, love/relationships, money/finances, life purpose/career. See where you need help—asking for help is NOT weak! It shows tremendous courage and strength!! Insanity is trying the same thing over and over without having a changed outcome! Ask for help and watch your life transform!

8. **Dance, jump rope, exercise**—this clears your energy field and releases endorphins, the pain-relieving chemical.

- Exercise raises your energy levels and opens the door for positive things to happen in your life. When people have low energy and are tired, they tend to stay in a rut or even have a downward spiral.

9. **Do what you love.**

- Cultivate a hobby, do what you love and say no to the things that don't light you up. Your time is precious, and each day we can create a life that excites us!

10. **Use Essential Oils.**

- Essential oils are topical and natural, and they help raise your vibration. Using them on a daily basis helps keep your immune system strong and your emotions balanced.

All of these practices impact your energy and lighten you up!

Your personal energy field can be *light* or **heavy** depending on:

- Your personal daily choices and habits.
- The health of the environment you're in at work and at home.
- The thoughts and feelings you have about yourself and others.
- How judgmental you are of others.
- If you have a strong 'inner critic'.
- If you use guilt and shame to control other people.
- The foods/beverages you ingest.

We have talked about many of these items in this book, so you are aware of how to "lighten up" through nutrition, thoughts you think, dropping judgments and taking your power back. As you shift each of these items listed above, you will notice an inner shift that leads to permanent change. This is way different than simply trying a new "diet" or shake. You are changing your energy from the inside out and will be able to carry this with you for the rest of your life!

Understanding Your Personal Energy System

Through my personal journey, I noticed that for much of my life I stayed in fearful thought patterns that were perpetuating my eating disorder. I knew that something needed to change internally in order to heal. When I came across the chakra (energy) system, I found there were other patterns I needed to break.

I was so afraid to speak my truth, especially in the face of a male authority figure. I never wanted to rock the boat for fear of having someone withdraw from me. Relationships with guys were hot and cold—I would get very close to them and then push them away because I couldn't trust myself. I wanted the certainty of love in my life, but I couldn't trust myself to choose the right people to give it. I also thought I was unworthy so I attracted unavailable men, which confirmed me not being worthy.

Perpetuating the same pattern means there is a core belief that creates an emotion in your body and will attract the same type of circumstance over and over until you learn the lesson. Ignoring an illness and masking symptoms with prescription drugs will never heal you. The same goes for unhealthy relationship patterns. Something is motioning for you to pay attention to heal the underlying belief. There may be energy blocks and limiting beliefs within you that prevent you from healing core wounds from childhood.

Healer Caroline Myss speaks about how our energies get taken in and are governed by the chakra system, which consists of 7 energy fields. Everyone has an energy field or aura that surrounds us and interpenetrates the physical body. This energy field is intimately associated with health.

Many times the source of illness comes from psychological or physical trauma or a combination of the two. Congested chakras reveal where the source of illness is.

Every chakra acts to vitalize each auric body and thus the physical body. The chakras are each associated with a major endocrine gland and nerve plexus. For example, the first chakra is associated with the adrenals, which deal with stress hormones such as cortisol and adrenaline. If this area is congested, a person may experience a multitude of symptoms such as ADHD, acne, or an autoimmune disease such as psoriasis, rheumatoid arthritis, etc.

When a chakra is energized and balanced, it will exhibit a clear, vibrant color in the energy field and will rotate evenly in a clockwise direction. A congested chakra will have a dull hue in the energy field and may be stagnant or rotating counter-clockwise if undercharged.

Functions of the Chakra System:

Chakra	Endocrine Function	Area of Body Governed	When balanced	When blocked, either excessive or deficient
1	Adrenals	Kidneys, spine	Strong will to live, grounded, feeling safe	Acne, arthritis, autoimmune diseases, constipation Excessive: overly possessive; fearful parent Deficient: homeless; ungrounded; victim
2	Gonads	Reproductive system	Ability to express emotions, Sense of abundance and well-being, Healthy sexual function	Fertility problems, urinary problems, hip/pelvic/low back pain Excessive: manipulative, controlling, lustful, addictive Deficient: co-dependent, martyr, submissive, doesn't feel anything, shut down
3	Pancreas	Gallbladder, stomach, liver	Self-worth, confidence, esteem, clear thinking	Digestive problems, diabetes, eating disorders, controlling/critical behavior Excessive: egotistical, self-absorbed; ambitious self-driven warrior, desire to take control Deficient: poor self-worth; sensitive servant; feels disliked; martyr; needing to "do" all the time
4	Thymus	Heart, blood, circulatory system	Love, ability to forgive, joy and inner peace	Congestive Heart failure, anger, bitterness Excessive: inappropriate emotional expression; poor emotional boundaries Deficient: ruthless, no heart, can't feel emotions

5	Thyroid	Bronchial and vocal apparatus, lungs	Self-expression, speaking the truth	Under/overactive Thyroid, TMJ, ADHD, neck/shoulder pain, ulcers Excessive: willful, controlling, judgmental, hurtful speech Deficient: lacking faith, unable to creatively express, silent child
6	Pituitary	Ears, nose, nervous system, lower brain	Clear thinking and decision-making, intuition	Migraines/headaches, blurred vision, hearing loss Excessive: overly intellectual; overly analytical Deficient: unclear thought; deluded
7	Pineal	Upper brain	Pure bliss, self-knowledge and divine connection	Confusion, fear of alienation Excessive: cult leader, ego maniac Deficient: no spiritual inspiration/aspiration

If your answer is YES to any of the following questions, you may be blocked or have a congested chakra in the corresponding energy center:

1. **Root Chakra** –Do you feel stuck in your current life situation? Did you recently have a traumatic event, family problems, death of a loved one, or other major life change?
2. **Sacral Chakra** – Do you feel unmotivated for life especially exercise or sex? Do you have an addiction or eating disorder? Low libido?
3. **Solar Plexus Chakra** – Do you have a sugar addiction, eating disorder or insomnia? How well do you set boundaries with others?
4. **Heart Chakra** – Do you feel disconnected to yourself and others with an inability to love? Do you feel that love is hopeless?
5. **Throat Chakra** – Do you have attention deficit disorder? Feel isolated, nervous/anxious? How well do you speak your truth?

6. **Third Eye Chakra** – Do you have trouble making decisions and feel confused and unable to follow your intuition?

7. **Crown Chakra** – Do you feel disconnected spiritually and that you cannot find your direction or purpose?

For example, a 3rd chakra imbalance comes from lack of healthy boundaries, meaning you typically say "yes" when you mean "no," betraying your true feelings. I used to do this because I felt so guilty saying no to people. I had weak boundaries, and no power.

Many people are caregivers/healers and are selfless people! It is a beautiful thing to be selfless and serve others. However, there needs to be an energy exchange, a giving, and receiving. Often people-pleasers will have the mentality that they need to help others before helping themselves. Think about it, how can you serve and give to others if you are depleted? I liken it to the airplane oxygen mask—you are supposed to put on your own mask before putting it over the child or other person you are with.

Other people lose energy from constant anger and frustration because they are resistant to what is in the present moment. These are the people you see screaming at customer service or exploding at their spouse for something insignificant. When you resist life, you create pain, which blocks life-force energy and ultimately leads to disease. This is a 1st chakra block along with a 7th. You are unwilling to accept the present moment, to feel connected to the earth and a higher power.

Accepting the present moment and realizing that the only thing we can control is how we respond is the way to let go of anger. You can feel the anger and release it, but if you do not process it you, will project it. Also, blaming and lack of forgiveness blocks energy and leaves you powerless. This is a 4th chakra block in the heart center. Taking ownership and responsibility of your part in the situation does not excuse bad behavior of others, but allows you to take your power back.

When you blame others for your pain, you are acting out the role of a victim. Seeing illness as a gift and opportunity to correct the imbalances in your life will allow you to heal.

Many caregivers and mothers wind up having a 3rd chakra imbalance from giving too much and not having balance of care for others and care for self. I have worked with many people who give too much of themselves, so much that they forget about taking care of themselves. They are unable to set healthy limits on how much of themselves they give to a project for their boss or the needs of their child, and they wind up suppressing or ignoring their own needs. Or, as in many eating-disorder cases, people seek approval from others to be validated for their own self-worth.

If you don't set healthy limits with people, your energy will be drained. There is a way to do this so that you do not feel guilty or feel like you are hurting the other person. Take ownership of your feelings and do not project. For example, if you are feeling tired and want to leave the table at dinner, you could say something like, "Listen, I'm feeling tired and need to excuse myself. I'll catch up with you later." It sounds simple, but for someone who is not used to setting boundaries and honoring their feelings and body, this is tremendous for energy conservation. This is a way to take care of yourself.

How to Align Your Energy Centers (Chakras):

1. Encourage positive thought patterns.
2. Get out in the sun for a few hours.
3. Eat foods that contain each of the seven color energies.
4. Do meditation and yoga.
5. Wear gemstones or place them in your environment.

6. Practice aromatherapy. My favorite is lavender and sandalwood.
7. Listen to music and dance.
8. Listen to high vibrational toning & sounds like Tibetan Bowls or gongs. **See Appendix C – Revitalize: Energy Practices.**
9. Color Tonations: shine light through various color filters over a specific area of the body.
10. Decorate your home or office with positive colors; surround yourself with color (calming colors in bedroom, stimulating colors in workplace.)
11. Receive a Reiki or massage treatment.

When you align your chakra system, you will feel revitalized and energetic!

Are You Ready for Radical Self-Care?

Self-care refers to nourishing our physical, mental, emotional, and spiritual well-being through various activities or practices. Self-care involves taking time out for yourself to recharge your physical body. Meditating, watching a funny video on YouTube to ease tension, going for a drive and getting lost in the din of the music, watching the clouds drift by—these are all acts of self-care. Whatever activities resonate with you are the ones you can stick to and repeat as often as you'd like.

Many of us have grown up hearing phrases like "Don't be selfish" or "You are a good person if you take care of others first." There is a huge misconception that self-care is equivalent to selfishness since we are prioritizing our needs and may have to take time away from other plans in our day. However, to love and serve others, we must first tend to ourselves. This is why self-care is so important. It's difficult for us to truly give our attention, love, and care to others when we are depleted. Taking the time to rejuvenate ourselves through these practices allows our energy to become amplified with a current of presence, or aliveness.

We all need self-care, especially during times of high stress. Stress cuts us off from creativity, while self-care renews it. When we are in balance, removed from stress and are happy, we can then fully give our awareness to those we love, creating harmony in this world.

What are some examples of self-care practices?

Spiritual:

- Cultivate a meditation practice.
- Make time for family/friends.
- Make time for reflection.
- Spend time in nature.
- Contribute to causes that you believe in.
- Read inspirational literature or listen to inspirational talks.

Psychological:

- Create a plan to reduce stress as much as possible.
- Practice receiving from others.
- Write in a journal.
- Be curious.
- Notice your inner experience: listen to your thoughts, judgments, beliefs, attitudes, and feelings.
- Say no to extra responsibilities when you feel overwhelmed.
- Stop gossiping and complaining.

Physical:

- Get a monthly massage.

- Reiki energy healing.
- Hot yoga, dancing, walking with a friend.
- Prepare healthy meals for yourself.
- Take the proper supplementation to support mental/physical health.
- Take time off and vacations when needed.
- Get enough sleep (7-9 hours a night).
- Take time to be sexual/experience pleasure.

Emotional:

- Discover what you did right and jot it down in your gratitude journal.
- Find things that make you laugh.
- Allow yourself to cry for 5-10 minutes and release the energy instead of resisting it.
- Seek out comforting people, activities, and places.

In the Workplace:

- Take regular breaks when needed.
- Socialize and connect with peers/colleagues.
- Balance your workload so it is not overburdening you.
- Speak up when you need help.

When we don't take care of ourselves, we get sick. This happened to me in March of 2018 after I had traveled to New York twice and then to Washington D.C. I went home to see my parents in January, went to a 5 day hypnosis training in February and volunteered at Landmark in March. The volunteering required 16 hours of our time each day. Although I was fulfilled and had gained so much from the experience, by the end of it, I was drained.

I hit the ground running after Landmark with networking meetings, writing blogs, meeting with nutrition and hypnosis clients and getting back to my boot camp classes. When I got sick, I was frustrated. I thought to myself, "What a time to get sick! I have so much to do." Little did I realize how smart my body was. It was screaming, "Take a break! Stop and relax!"

The flu lasted 5 days, and I had a chance to relax with very minimal work or demands on me. Sometimes our body nudges us with signals like a headache or tension in our upper back. However, if we just override those signals, we become sick.

Take small steps each day to take care of yourself and to tune into your energy. Are you feeling tense? Frustrated? Where are you daily on the scale of consciousness? If you find that you are below Courage, ask yourself 'How can I raise my energy to a good feeling place?' Self-care activities can certainly help you get there.

No matter what you go through in your day-to-day experience, there is always an empowered way to look at something. There is a lesson in everything you go through. Even if it is challenging or it seems hopeless, I encourage you to look at the silver lining and see what you are learning in that moment.

If you are sick, do you need to set better boundaries and have more time for yourself?

If you are going through a rough breakup, how can you take the best care of yourself and find a positive meaning in what you've learned from that relationship? What beliefs can you let go of?

If you feel dejected by failed diet attempts, what action steps can you glean from this book to put into place?

In challenging times, always look for the lesson and how you can grow from that experience. In good times, relish every moment and enjoy! Life is meant to be enjoyed. Soak up every moment!

Reflection Week 7

1. How can you increase your self-care routine in the next 30 days?
   ➢ Emotionally
   ➢ Mentally
   ➢ Physically
   ➢ Spiritually

2. What is getting in the way of you raising your frequency to a good feeling place? Think of habits you have that are getting in the way of moving you up the scale of consciousness. Some examples are gossiping, criticizing, cursing, negative self-talk and judging.

3. From the chakra chart, where might you have imbalances? What tools resonated with you to realign your energy system?

Dr. Christina Tarantola

Throughout this book I've highlighted several ways to nourish your body, mind, and spirit through nutrition, shifting your belief system, recharging and letting go of the past. My team of pharmacists has done a phenomenal job, in **Appendix C**, of listing out powerful techniques you can utilize to keep the momentum with your new habits. Practices like sound healing, Reiki, meditation, vision boards, affirmations, and gratitude will augment the work you've done so far and keep you feeling good!

As you continue on in your life and see the transformation, offer this book to someone else who can use it. If we simply learn something and apply it, it certainly helps us. However, if we *share* our experience and allow others to create their own experience, it is even more powerful. This is how we create change in our community and in our world.

With love and gratitude,
Christina

Appendix

Appendix

Appendix A: Healing Your Gut For Optimal Health

The health of your gastrointestinal tract (GIT) is significant for maintaining overall health. Your gut plays an important role not only in regulating digestion but also in supporting your immune system, synthesizing neurotransmitters such as serotonin, regulating mineral and vitamin absorption, supporting elimination and controlling hormones. Many inflammatory conditions can arise from "leaky gut syndrome," a condition where the integrity of the lining of the GI tract is compromised, and foreign particles seep out into your bloodstream, raising the alarm bells for your immune system. Sounds pleasant, doesn't it?!

Maintaining a healthy GIT is paramount!

Here are some of my favorite supplements and foods to help support the integrity of your gut:

1. **Collagen.** Collagen is the most abundant protein in our bodies, especially type 1 collagen. It's found in muscles, bones, skin, blood vessels, digestive system, and tendons. It's what helps give our skin strength and elasticity, along with replacing dead skin cells. When it comes to our joints and tendons, in simplest terms, it's the "glue" that helps hold the body together.

   As we age, collagen production decreases. Lifestyle factors such as smoking, consuming a diet high in sugar and excessive sun exposure can also contribute to a decrease in collagen. Supplementing daily can help support your joints, skin elasticity, and digestive health.

Brand I recommend: Vital Proteins powder – Amazon

Use daily in a hot beverage such as tea or coffee, as a substitute for protein powder or in recipes.

2. **Bone broth.** If collagen had a brother, bone broth would be his name. Bone broth is made from...bones. If you have ever had chicken soup when you were sick, this was why. Bone broth can help heal leaky gut syndrome, boost immunity, improve skin health and overcome food intolerances.

Brand I recommend: Ancient Nutrition – turmeric, vanilla or chocolate flavors or EPIC – beef jalapeno sea salt, home-style savory chicken, bison apple cider, turkey cranberry sage.

Making your own bone broth:

[Modified recipe from herbalist Claudia Keel, www.EarthFlower.org]

Ingredients:

- Chicken bones (roasted or raw) including cartilage parts, found in neck, feet, and head. Seek out organic, pastured poultry — the higher quality ingredients, the higher quality the stock.
- Apple Cider Vinegar or any acid – such as lemon juice
- Water - filtered or spring
- Optional: chicken meat and/or gizzards (organs)
- Additional herbs and vegetables: bay leaves, thyme, sage, peppercorns, carrots, celery, parsley, garlic and onion, ginger

Recipe:

1. Combine the chicken bones, parts and other ingredients in a large stockpot or crockpot, along with apple cider vinegar (1/4 cup for every 4-6 quarts) and enough cold water to cover the ingredients. Let sit for 1 hour off heat to increase the amount of gelatin and minerals released from the bones.
2. Bring to a boil and skim the scum that comes to the top. (These are impurities and off flavors. Organic pasture-raised poultry will have much less scum). Then turn down to a simmer, and cover. Simmer on low for 12 to 48 hours. If using the crockpot, turn to low and let cook for 12 to 48 hours.
3. In the hour before finishing, add green herbs, salt, and pepper.
4. Allow to cool, and strain into a glass jar for storage.
5. Put in the refrigerator for up to five days or in the freezer for several months. Be careful when freezing liquids in glass jars, as there is a risk of breaking the jar. Minimize the risk by keeping the level of liquid below the shoulder of the jar and not capping tightly until frozen. Or opt for other freezer storage containers, preferably BPH-free such as silicone or stainless steel.

3. **Fermented foods.** These are foods that are left to steep until the sugars and carbohydrates become bacteria-boosting agents. They are rich in probiotics and support the normal flora in your GI tract. Fermented foods lead to an increase in digestive function and immunity, as well as help to regulate appetite and reduce cravings.
Foods I recommend: Pickled foods and lacto-fermented foods such as kimchi, sauerkraut, kombucha, kefir, yogurt, and tempeh. Fermented foods
Supplements I recommend: Each probiotic strain can have different effects such as regulating hormones or enhance immune function. Look for a high CFU (colony forming unit) with at least 15 billion active cultures. Make sure to look for a variety of different strains such as Bifidobacterium, Lactobacillus, and Sacchromyces.

Do some research and ensure that the strains in your probiotic are supporting your needs.

4. **High fiber foods.** If probiotics are the nail, fiber is the sledgehammer. Fiber helps probiotics thrive in the gut, and assists in productive bowel movements.

    Foods to incorporate: Chia seeds, flaxseed, and steamed vegetables are some examples of high fiber foods.

5. **DGL (deglycyrrhizinated licorice).** DGL is an adaptogenic herb, which means that it is derived from a unique class of healing plants and supports mitigating the stress response. DGL can help maintain the mucosal lining of the stomach and reduces inflammation.

    Licorice normally contains glycyrrhizin, which can cause water retention and increase in blood pressure in some individuals. Deglycyrrhizinated licorice has that component removed to prevent additional side effects.

    Brand I recommend: Enzymatic Therapy DGL

    ***Disclaimer**: Before you start any new vitamin, supplement, herb, food, please check with your doctor or healthcare professional to ensure that there are no interactions or potential harmful effects.

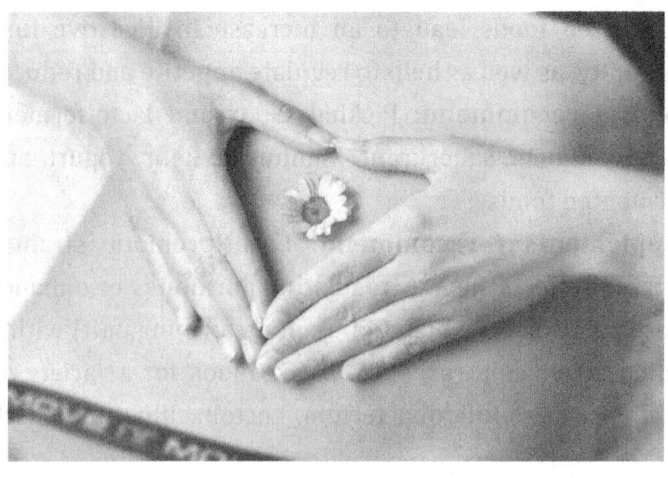

Gut Health

[Excerpt from Dr. Marina's expanded article at RawFork.com]

One of the most important things you can do for your health involves an organ system that technically doesn't touch the inside of your body. I'm talking about the gut, or the gastrointestinal tract (GIT). The length of this canal if unfolded outside the body is about seven times as long as a person's body, the majority of which is the small intestine! The food we ingest is converted each step of the way into a form that can be absorbed inside the body into a usable form, while the unusable mass is effectively eliminated.

In recent years, the discovery of the 'microbiome' revealed that there is more bacteria living inside an individual's gut than there are human cells! That's a whole new perspective on what is considered a 'human' and where we end and 'non-self' begins. The bacteria perform a variety of functions vital to our health and survival.

Also, the gut houses the enteric nervous system (ENS), which is known as 'the second brain.' Neurotransmitters such as serotonin and dopamine influence digestion as well as your mood! This connection is implicated in frequent bouts of diarrhea when a person is nervous, or depression/anxiety when the gut is not working properly. Now you know that your 'gut feeling,' 'butterflies in your stomach' has a physiological basis, and you can learn to tune in on these messages from your body!

I consider the gut the foundation of physical and emotional health, and always look to it first when consulting clients. Its role is critical in converting 'not-self' to 'self,' to absorbing vital nutrients, optimizing immunity and communicating with the nervous system. I have personally been a victim of and witness to many symptoms and syndromes that ultimately tie back to gut integrity, and I'm passionate about spreading that message to others. I believe if you can heal your gut, you can heal your life.

I'd like to review the organs that make up the gut and how you can optimize the function of each.

1. **The mouth.** Here digestion officially begins both by mechanically (chewing) and chemically (amylase enzyme). While the enzyme content can't really be helped, we can certainly work on the physical grinding action of our teeth.

   - Eating mindfully by taking smaller bites and chewing slowly and deliberately helps reduce particle size of food for easier digestion in the rest of the tract.

   - Ayurvedic tradition focuses on the tongue as an organ that represents the health of the person and his/her digestive power. To help the entire system work better, cleaning the tongue with a copper or stainless steel cleaner is recommended.

   - Coconut oil 'pulling' is also thought to improve the cleanliness of mouth, improve dental hygiene and thus improve the state of health of the gut. To do this: place ½ - 1 teaspoon of coconut oil in mouth first thing in the morning, and try to 'thread' it in between each tooth as if you're flossing with the oil, then spit into trash can (oils can clog plumbing systems!) and brush as usual.

2. **The esophagus.** This tube connects the mouth to the stomach and is separated by the lower esophageal sphincter (LES) from the stomach. The LES is a circular group of muscles that opens and closes to make a one-way tract down into the stomach, thus preventing backflow of the acidic content back up the esophagus. Problems can arise when the LES is weakened and

the acid escapes, which can erode the mucosa of the esophagus and throat, resulting in gastroesophageal reflux disease (GERD).

- Foods to avoid in order to prevent weakening the LES: caffeine (coffee, chocolate), alcohol, peppermint.

- Not lying down or reclining after meals should ensure the correct flow of peristalsis and prevent reflux.

- Sleeping with an incline from the waist up can also help keep acid down where it belongs.

3. **The stomach.** Here hydrochloric acid (HCl) and enzymes (pepsin) help chemically break down the chewed food particles as well as defend against potential pathogens. The optimal gastric pH level is 1-2. The danger of the pH being too low is eroding the mucosal layer surrounding the stomach, which can cause ulcers and potentially deadly bleeding. A low pH is also associated with the bacterial overgrowth and with the development of ulcers.

- Conventional medicine treats this problem by lowering the production of acid, which can lead to other problems down the line, from infections to osteoporosis.

- Alternative treatments of GERD are herbal bitters, which enhance digestion and help liver detox. Examples include dandelion root, gentian root, and artichoke leaf.

- Sometimes the symptoms presenting as GERD are actually due to low stomach acid, which presents due to a feedback mechanism that lowers the amount of protective mucous lining around the stomach. Here are some things you can do to help normalize acid levels:

- o   Eating smaller meals and chewing mindfully.

- o   Taking apple cider vinegar or HCl with pepsin supplement before meals, or digestive enzymes during meals.

4. **The small intestine.** This is the longest part of the GI, measuring about 3.5 times of a person's height! Despite being narrow in diameter, if entirely unfolded and unfurled, its surface area would be about the size of a tennis court. This anatomy allows the small intestine to absorb all the digested nutrients into the bloodstream via 'tight gap junctions' in the fingerlike projections along its walls. Remember when I said that technically the 'gut' is outside our bodies? Well, the small intestine is what determines what we can assimilate from the outside in. Many problems can arise in this step of the digestive process.

    - •   Intestinal hyperpermeability, or 'leaky gut': is a major cause of allergies and autoimmunity, and an array of chronic inflammatory, degenerative and neurological conditions (anything from inflammatory bowel diseases, Parkinson's disease, depression/anxiety, migraines, autism to coronary artery disease, diabetes, and cancer). If the gap junctions are not tight enough, they become 'leaky' and allow in particles that normally should not be present in our bloodstreams. This can set off a whole chain of hypersensitivity reactions leading not only to allergies but to autoimmune issues down the line. To heal 'leaky gut', we must repair the integrity of the gap junctions via:

        - o   The GAPS (Gut and Psychology Syndrome) diet

- o Collagen consumed in the form of food (bone broth) or supplement (collagen or gelatin)

- o Anti-inflammatory diet and supplements

- IBS (Irritable Bowel Syndrome): a group of symptoms consisting of bloating/gas, abdominal cramps, and bouts of constipation/diarrhea. Also, depression and anxiety are common comorbidities, which is related to the gut-brain connection. The following can help balance the disorder:

  - o Avoid inflammatory foods and allergens such as dairy, wheat/gluten, soy, eggs, caffeine, alcohol, processed foods, sugar, and FODMAPs (Fermentable Oligosaccharides, Disaccharides, Monosaccharides, and Polyols).

  - o Reduce stress by mindfulness practices and exercise.

  - o Supplements to consider:
    - Pro- and prebiotics
    - Aloe vera
    - L-glutamine
    - Adaptogenic herbs (licorice)
    - Digestive enzymes or carminative herbs (fennel, chamomile, orange peel) to help with bloating/indigestion
    - Anti-inflammatory supplements such as omega-3 fish oil

- SIBO (Small Intestine Bacterial Overgrowth): a condition where bacteria normally present in the large intestine colonizes part of the small intestine. This causes uncomfortable bloating and gas after eating almost anything, as well as malabsorption of nutrients - due to bacterial fermentation of food particles. While conventional therapy aims to kill the excess bacteria via antibiotics, a holistic approach to SIBO includes:

- o First decrease the amount of fermentable foods, such as the FODMAPs diet for a few weeks; then initiate GAPS or SCD (Specific Carbohydrate Diet) protocol to heal the integrity of the gut.

- o Eat smaller, more frequent meals.

- o Supplement with probiotics to restore proper microbiome.

- o Herbal bitters

5. **The large intestine.** The final step of digestion involves reabsorbing all the water and salts that were not usable as nutrients via the small intestine. This water combines with waste material (fiber from food, bile acids, dead cells from intestine lining) to be passed as formed stool. Also, this is the site of the microbiome - the vastly diverse bacterial colonies that help absorb certain vitamins (such as B12), digest fiber, detox certain substances (such as drugs) and ferment the leftover food matter into passable gases. Symptoms of imbalance usually present as constipation/diarrhea or pain.

- To prevent constipation, stay hydrated and include fiber in your diet (fruit and vegetable peels, plums, prunes, beets). Also, avoid constipating foods like starches or grains, pears, and bananas.

- Taking antibiotics can throw off the natural flora of the colon and may make it more vulnerable to be populated by opportunistic pathogens resulting in acute inflammation (colitis).

o The more diverse the bacterial species are, the healthier the body! Probiotics help optimize the microbiome and are an absolute must for someone taking antibiotics. Natural sources of probiotics include fermented foods such as sauerkraut, kimchi, kefir or yogurt.

o Prebiotics (indigestible sugars that feed the microbiome) are also important, and are contained in starchy roots vegetables and herbs. Some probiotic supplements already contain this in their formula as 'inulin.'

• IBD (Inflammatory Bowel Disease) such as ulcerative colitis (UC) or the more severe Crohn's disease (CD) is an inflammatory condition that erodes the lining of the colon.

o Conventional treatment focuses on an array of inflammation-suppressing medications, whereas holistic approaches target the hypothesized cause of the immune overreaction, using the same approach as for 'leaky gut.' Eating a 'traditional diet' of three large meals a day with plenty of good fats and proteins, and bone broth can be very helpful in slowing bowel movements and healing the mucosa.

Appendix B: Healing Through Nutrition Recipes

The core principles of the way these meals are formatted were adapted from The Diet Doc book, *50 Days to Your Best Life!* My study of science-based nutrition under Dr. Joe Klemczewski inspired me to write this section of the book.

These recipes are meant to provide you with sustained energy from whole food sources. If you need to adjust any of the recipes for your own dietary restrictions, please do so. I recommend you follow your own unique food preferences and what works for your body.

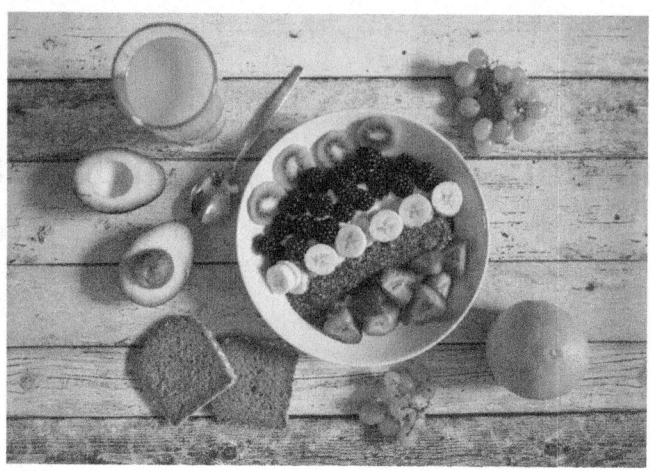

Breakfast

- Too big of a breakfast will cause an increase in insulin and create lethargy early in the morning.
- Too small of a breakfast will leave you feeling hungry early on in the day.
- Upon waking up, blood sugar and amino acid levels are low. Reversing this as soon as possible with breakfast is important to retain muscle and spur metabolism.

Protein/starch combinations for women:
- ½ cup (measured dry) oatmeal and 1 scoop protein powder
- 3 Egg whites and 1 whole grain 100 calorie English muffin
- ½ cup Greek yogurt or cottage cheese and 1 slice of whole grain toast
- ½ cup high fiber cereal and 4 egg whites

Protein/starch combinations for men:
- ½ cup (measured dry) oatmeal and 1 scoop protein powder
- 5 Egg whites and 1 whole grain 100 calorie English muffin

- 1 cup Greek yogurt or cottage cheese and 2 slices of whole grain toast
- ½ cup high fiber cereal and 4 egg whites

Peach Cobbler Overnight Oats

Ingredients:
- ½ cup old fashioned oats
- ½ cup milk of your choice
- ¼ cup Greek yogurt
- ½ teaspoon ground cinnamon
- ¼ teaspoon ground nutmeg
- ½ cup diced peaches

Directions:
- Add all ingredients into glass jar or Tupperware with lid and stir until fully combined. Add peach slices on top and close the lid.
- Place in the refrigerator for at least 8 hours or overnight.
- Enjoy the next day!

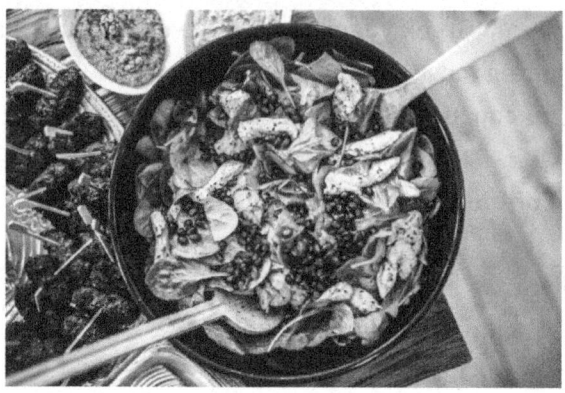

Lunch

- While we do not want to create a low-carb environment throughout the entire day, there can be a benefit to have a span of time where carbohydrates are low.
- You can decide whether you'd like your lunch to be your anchor meal or vice versa depending on your schedule day to day.
- A heavy meal during the day may lead to lethargy or the desire to take a nap, which can be a challenge for people who need to work until the late afternoon!

Protein/Fiber combinations for women:
- 3 oz chicken breast, 2 cups of green beans, ½ oz low-fat feta cheese, small salad with 1tbsp balsamic
- ½ whole grain English muffin, 1 can of tuna in water and 1 oz avocado
- 3 oz salmon, 1 cup asparagus, ¼ cup cooked brown rice

Protein/Fiber combinations for men:
- 3 oz chicken breast, 1 oz fat-free cheese, 1 cup fresh spinach, ½ oz walnuts, 1 cup strawberries and 1 tbsp low-fat dressing

- 1 whole grain English muffin, 1 can of tuna in water, 1 oz avocado, 1 cup lettuce, 1 oz diced tomato, 2 boiled egg whites
- ½ cup plain Greek yogurt, ¼ cup high fiber cereal, ½ tsp flaxseed oil, ¾ scoop protein powder

For lunch, I like to make something light like cucumber, tomato and feta cheese with a drizzle of olive oil and some grilled chicken.

Greek Cucumber Dill Salad

Ingredients:
- 3 English cucumbers
- 1 tablespoon freshly chopped dill
- 1 garlic clove, minced
- 1 lemon, zested and juiced
- ½ cup plain Greek yogurt
- Salt and pepper

Directions:
- Peel the cucumbers. Cut in half lengthwise then slice into thin pieces. Place the sliced cucumbers into a large bowl.
- Add the chopped dill, minced garlic, zest of one lemon, 1 tbsp lemon juice, Greek yogurt, sugar, ½ teaspoon of salt and ¼ teaspoon ground black pepper.
- Toss until the yogurt blends into a thin dressing. Add salt and pepper to taste and serve cold.

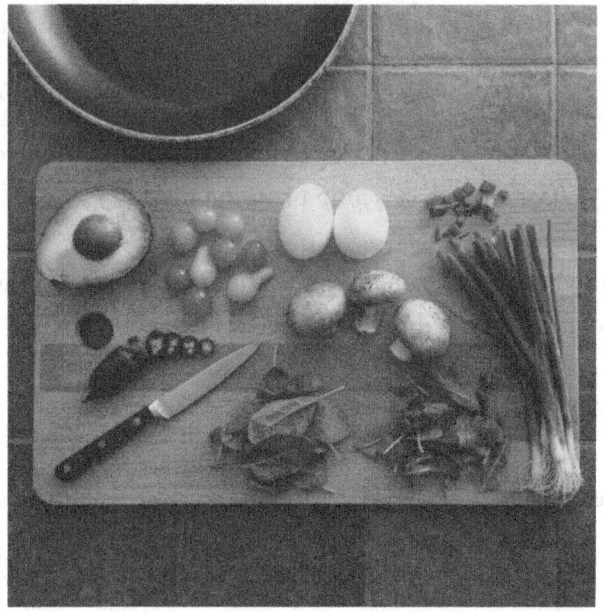

Dinner

- If too little is eaten, it can trigger eating late at night-a common breakdown of weight-loss programs.
- See picture below of the **MyPlateMethod**. ½ the plate is fibrous vegetables, ¼ of the plate is a lean protein and ¼ of the plate is a starchy carbohydrate.

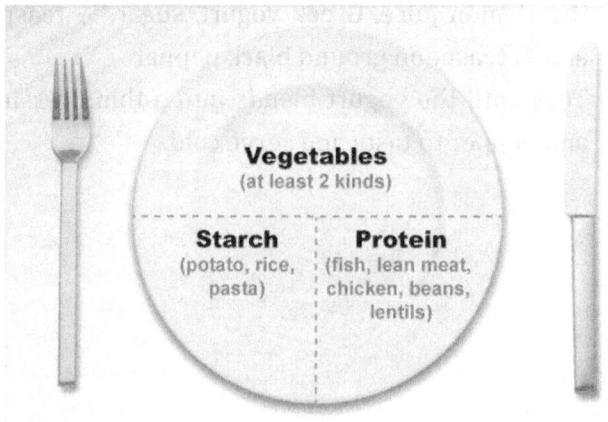

Protein/Starch/Fiber combinations for women:
- 1 small baked potato (5 oz), ½ cup low-fat cottage cheese, ¼ cup pizza sauce
- 2 oz shrimp, ½ cup of rice, ½ oz fat-free cheese, 1 oz spinach, 2 oz strawberries, 1 tbsp fat-free balsamic.
- 2 oz sirloin, 2 cups broccoli, 3 oz potato

Protein/Starch/Fiber combinations for men:
- 4 oz chicken breast, ½ cup chunky marinara, 1 cup butternut squash, 3 oz sautéed onions/zucchini
- 4 oz salmon, 1 cup cooked rice noodles, 1 cup broccoli, 1 tbsp parmesan cheese
- 1 cup skim milk, 1 cup cereal, ¼ cup blueberries, ¾ scoop protein powder, 1 tbsp flaxseeds

Pre-workout meals:
- You want to have simple carbohydrates right before a workout (20-30 minutes) so that your body's energy is not being used for digestion instead of fueling your workout.
- If you have a larger snack, have it at least an hour before you workout so you are not full and trying to digest while you exercise.
- 15-20 grams of carbohydrates will suffice for a pre-workout snack.

Examples for women include:
- 1 rice cake, 1 tbsp jam, 1 tsp peanut butter
- ½ banana and 1 tsp peanut butter
- ¼ cup oats and 2 oz blueberries

Examples for men include:
- 2 rice cakes, 2tbsp jam, ½ tbsp peanut butter

- ¼ cup oats (dry measure), 2 oz blueberries
- 1 medium banana and ½ tbsp. peanut butter

Post-workout meals:

- For proper muscle recovery and anabolism (building), protein is the perfect solution. Cortisol levels are high after a workout, so adding protein can blunt that effect. Adding carbohydrates to a post-workout meal can help recovery and muscle growth as well, especially after a cardio workout.

Examples for women include:

- ½ scoop protein powder, 1/8 serving high fiber cereal
- 4 egg whites, 1 low-carb tortilla
- ½ cup plain Greek yogurt, 1 oz blueberries and ¼ oz chopped nuts

Examples for men include:

- 3 oz chicken breast and ½ mini bagel
- 1 scoop protein powder in water and 1 rice cake
- 4 oz extra lean ground beef, ¼ cup cooked rice

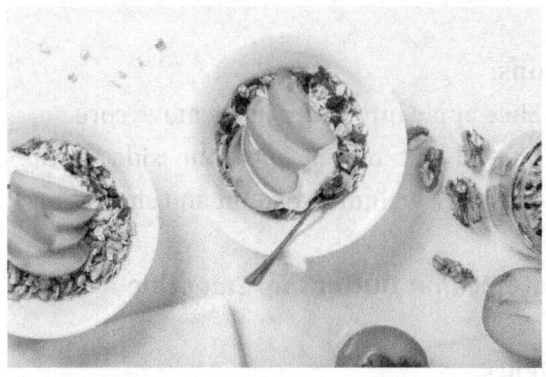

Snack

(1/2 serving of protein and starch):

- This can be a snack at any point during the day OR if you go to bed much later at night and you eat dinner early.

Examples for women include:

- 1 slice light bread, ½ tbsp. peanut butter
- ½ banana, ½ tbsp. peanut butter
- ½ apple and 1 piece light string cheese

Examples for men include:

- 1 slice whole-grain bread, ½ tbsp. peanut butter
- 2 rice cakes and ¼ cup fat-free cottage cheese
- ½ cup low-fat yogurt

Apple cookies

Ingredients:

- 1 apple
- ¼ cup peanut butter or almond butter
- ¼ cup almonds, sliced
- ¼ cup walnuts, chopped
- ¼ cup shredded coconut
- ¼ cup chocolate chips or cacao nibs

Directions:
- Slice apple into rings and remove core
- Spread nut butter over one side of the ring. Top with almonds, walnuts, coconut and chocolate chips.

Chocolate Peanut Butter Cup Smoothie

Ingredients:
- 3/4 cup unsweetened almond milk
- 1 scoop of your favorite chocolate protein powder
- 2 tablespoons powdered peanut butter
- 1 large slightly ripened banana, cubed and frozen

Directions:
- Add all ingredients to blender and mix on high speed until blended. Serve immediately.

Raspberry Frozen Yogurt Bites

Ingredients:
- ¼ cup crushed almonds or almond meal
- 2 tablespoons coconut sugar
- 2 tablespoons coconut oil, melted
- ¾ cup plain 0% Greek yogurt
- 2 tablespoons honey
- 1 ½ cups freshly chopped strawberries and/or raspberries
- 6 cup muffin tin and liners

Directions:
- Line the muffin tin with silicone or parchment cupcake liners
- In a small bowl, stir together crushed almonds, coconut

sugar, and coconut oil. Spoon a small amount into each muffin cup.

- In a medium bowl, mix together yogurt and honey. Spoon 2 tablespoons into each muffin cup, covering the crust.
- Top with berries. Freeze until firm, about 6 hours. To serve, remove from silicone wrapper and allow to sit at room temperature for 8-10 minutes.

Appendix C: Revitalize—Energy Practices

These energy practices are meant to help enhance your journey throughout the 7 weeks. When our energy is out of alignment, we can get sick, the body gets out of balance and we feel "off." Utilizing these practices will help you revitalize and gain clarity and focus to master your health.

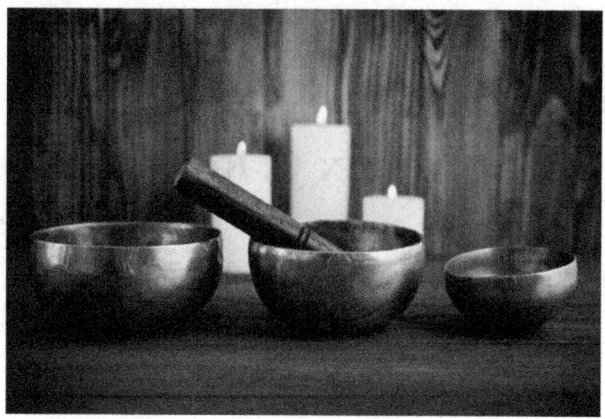

Sound Healing

Sound is considered an ancient form of healing. Since everything in the world is made up of energy, the presence of disease alters the vibration of the body. Resonance is the frequency at which an object naturally vibrates. Each part of our bodies has it's own natural resonance, and vibrational medicine is based on the idea that disease is a result of those natural resonances getting out of tune due to stress, illness or environmental factors.

Sound can reduce the effects of the stress hormone cortisol, slow heart rate and improve immunity. Sound therapy works to restore balance to the body and remove energy blockages.

Sound helps to facilitate shifts in our brainwave state by using entrainment. Entrainment synchronizes our fluctuating brainwaves by providing a stable frequency, which the brainwave can attune to. Entrainment music therapy is described as *"any stimuli that matches or models the current mood state of the individual and then moves the person in the direction of a more positive or pleasant mood state."*

This is accomplished by shifting our brain waves from waking consciousness (beta wave) to a meditative state (theta waves). In

2008, the journal *Alternative Therapies in Health and Medicine* published a review of 20 studies of brain-wave entrainment and patient outcomes. The conclusion was that brain-wave entrainment is an effective tool to use on cognitive functioning deficits, stress, pain, headaches, and premenstrual syndrome.

Sound baths are an ancient healing technique that utilizes tools like Tibetan bowls, gongs, and tuning forks that emit sound at different frequencies to induce a meditative state.

Negative vibrations or high-pitched sounds can cause cells to mutate, while peaceful sounds restore normal structure of our DNA. A wide number of guided meditations are available online that use binaural tones which involve two different frequencies that create a harmonious frequency to bring the listener into a deep meditative state. At various frequencies, the body has the ability to heal through sound.

Solfeggio frequencies make up the ancient 6-tone scale used in sacred music, notably Gregorian Chants. These special tones were thought to impart spiritual blessings when sung in harmony. Each Solfeggio tone is comprised of a frequency required to balance your energy. The main 6 frequencies are:

1. 396 Hz – Liberating guilt and fear.
2. 417 Hz – Undoing situations and facilitating change.
3. 528 Hz – Transformation and miracles.
4. 639 Hz – Connecting and relationships.
5. 741 Hz – Expressions and solutions.
6. 852 Hz – Returning to spiritual order.

Here are some other examples of sound therapy:

Classical Music. Classical music has been shown to increase the rate of development of synaptic connections in young children's minds. It also helps fuel creativity and enhance joy in adults. Classical music can even help address physical ailments like high blood pressure and muscle tension.

Humming. Humming not only lifts your spirits, it clears your head. According to a study conducted by Swedish researcher, and published in the American Journal of Respiratory and Critical Care Medicine, humming may actually help keep your sinuses clear and healthy.

Singing Bowls. Whether metal or quartz crystal, a singing bowl sings when you run a felt-tipped mallet around its edge. Along with rhythms produced by striking the edge of the bowl, the vibrations and tones slow down breathing, brain waves and heart rates, producing a deep sense of calm and well-being.

Tuning Forks. Originally used to tune musical instruments to the proper pitch, tuning forks have long been used by orthopedists to detect stress fractures in large bones. Now, sound therapists use the vibrations of tuning forks to increase the amount of energy in parts of the body they are trying to heal or energize. These good vibes can support relaxation, balance our nervous systems and increase physical energy.

Yogic Chanting and "Om"ing. Chanting, the first step to meditation is also a means of maintaining health and well-being. Research shows that chanting can stabilize heart rate, lower blood pressure, improve circulation, produce endorphins and aid the process of metabolism. Chanting can also help the mind focus, which alleviates stress levels. For example, repeating the syllable "om," considered one of the most important mantras in yoga, is said to foster a deep mental clarity and promote a sense of connectedness with a higher power.

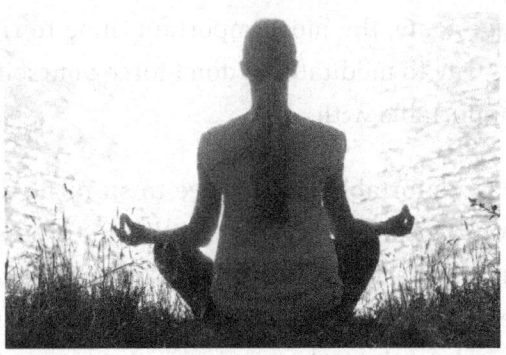

Meditation

With all the hustle and bustle of our daily lives, the practice of meditation has recently gained popularity and attention as a tool for mindfulness. With all that is demanded of us on a daily basis (jobs, family, social life, and other stresses) our brains are working overtime. How often do you find yourself saying, "I don't have time for that!", especially when it comes to taking care of yourself? You may be surprised at how taking a little time out of your day to meditate can change your whole perspective.

When you think of the word "meditation," you may think of an old, wise yogi, sitting cross-legged on a cushion, perfectly peaceful. While this interpretation isn't wrong, it conjures up the notion that there is a right and wrong way to meditate, which is not true. Meditation is essentially a practice of mindfulness – the idea of being mentally present, appreciating the "now," and being aware of your thoughts. It may sound simple, but sometimes we forget to stop and smell the roses because we are always worried about the future and what's coming next. There is an old Zen saying that goes, *"You should sit in meditation for 20 minutes a day unless you're too busy, then you should sit for an hour."*

Meditation allows you to spend some time just *being*, and there are many ways to practice this in your daily life:

Breathing: Again, the most important thing to remember is there is no "wrong" way to meditate, so don't force yourself to do something you're not comfortable with.

1. Find a comfortable, quiet place to sit or lie down. You can do this on a chair or cushion, with legs crossed or uncrossed, resting your arms gently on your knees or at your side.
2. Close your eyes, and breathe slowly and deeply through your nose and out through your mouth. Let your mind be still as you focus on your breathing. Allow yourself to notice the air filling your lungs, and as you exhale, imagine your worries and stress to be expelled with it. Sometimes, it helps to imagine a white or golden light entering your body from the top of your head.
3. If you catch your mind wandering, be mindful of this and let it go, and resume your practice of focusing on your body and breath. Set a timer and start small with 5 minutes. There are fantastic apps that help with guided meditation practices – check out "Headspace", "Insight Timer" and "Calm."

Loving-Kindness: This is a form of meditation that not only helps heal yourself but helps promote understanding and compassion for others. This technique has you repeat the mantra, *"May I feel safe, may I feel happy, may I live with ease."* You start with yourself, then extend it to others, using the word "you" instead of "I", and finally, repeating the mantra for the world. This selfless, loving form of meditation allows us to get out of our heads, stop focusing on our problems, and think of others. We can only send that pure type of love to others after it passes through us first, so it is possible that those of us who have a hard time loving or forgiving ourselves experience a kind of self-compassion we hadn't felt in a long time, and the healing becomes twofold.

Intentional Self-Care Time: Did you know that cooking yourself a healthy meal, taking a bubble bath, and listening to the sounds of nature are also all considered forms of meditation? Practicing self-care is a form of meditation because you become aware of your relaxation and unwinding. Reading self-help books or even just standing in the shower and paying attention to the feel of the water running down your body are meditative because your mind clears and focuses on the present moment. Find a method of self-care that works for you, as long as it raises your vibration instead of lowering it (see earlier in the chapter).

Meditation has a profound mental, emotional, and spiritual impact. Studies indicate that it is also beneficial for physical health. Meditation is useful for reducing anxiety and stress, which lowers disease risk. In one study from Harvard University, participants had magnetic resonance imaging (MRI) scans. After doing guided meditation, it was shown that they had experienced a thickening in the part of the brain (gray matter) responsible for emotions and perception. Such changes can strengthen the body's physiological resilience against worry, anxiety, and depression.

Another study found that it may increase the tone of the vagus nerve, which is the longest nerve in your body that starts in the brain and directly connects to every organ. The vagal tone is measured by tracking the difference in your heart rate as you breathe in and out. The greater the difference, the higher your vagal tone — which means the faster your body is able to relax after stress. High vagal tone is linked to better mood and lower risk of heart disease, while low vagal tone is linked to inflammation, negative moods, and increased stress.

Try to begin your meditative practice, whichever kind you choose, for even just five minutes a day, and see how it can improve your life. You will start to see the benefits in your mindset and your physical body!

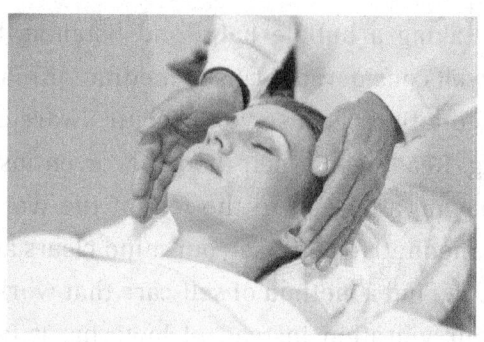

Reiki

Reiki is a Japanese spiritual healing ritual that involves the "laying on of hands." The word Reiki comes from the Japanese word "Rei" which refers to "Universal Life," and "Ki" which refers to energy.

Reiki is based on the Eastern principle that there is a "life-force" energy that flows through all living things. Reiki Practitioners believe that every person has the ability to connect with their own innate healing energy. A person's "ki" or energy should be strong and free-flowing; when this happens, a person's body and mind is in a positive state of health. When the energy becomes weak or blocked due to physical, mental, or emotion imbalance, it can lead to illness.

Mikao Usui, the founder of Reiki healing, developed The Five Ideals, or Five Principles. Consciously deciding to improve oneself is a necessary part of the Reiki healing experience. In order for the Reiki healing energies to have lasting results, the client must accept responsibility for her or his healing and take an active part in it. The Principles can be used as daily affirmations or mantras, even if you don't practice Reiki itself.

The Five Principles are:

- *Just for today, I will not worry.*

- *Just for today, I will not be angry.*
- *Just for today, I will be grateful.*
- *Just for today, I will do my work honestly.*
- *Just for today, I will be kind to every living thing."*

A Reiki session can help ease tension and stress and can help support the body to facilitate an environment for healing on all levels – physical, mental, and emotional. Reiki is performed in a calm environment, where the client lays down on a comfortable table. The room may be silent or might have gentle music playing. The practitioner will lay their hands over the client's body and work over the whole body to rebalance the chakra system. The session lasts anywhere between 30-60 minutes. The practitioner channels divine energy to the client to rebalance their energy system.

Some studies have shown that Reiki plays a positive role in promoting healing in patients with various conditions, especially used in conjunction with other forms of conventional and alternative medicine. Clients who have a more positive outlook in the face of a diagnosis will often have a better outcome and quality of life than clients who are negative and withdrawn.

The ability to use Reiki is not necessarily "taught," but is transferred through an attunement to a student during Reiki training. The "attunement" given by a Reiki master allows the student to tap into the life force energy to improve one's health and enhance the quality of life for others.

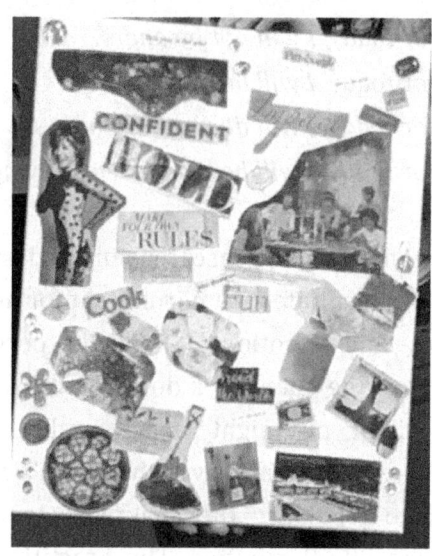

Visualization and Vision Boards

I have always been a visual learner and used to make vision boards as a little girl. Having a visual representation of what you want for your life triggers powerful subconscious pathways in your brain to discover new ways to achieve that goal. A vision board contains images that resonate with what you want to create in your life. Putting one together is a simple, fun way to capture the dreams you have for your life and have a constant reminder of what you want to manifest!

What exactly is a vision board? A vision board can be anything you want it to be. The idea is that it is a space for you to place an order for exactly what you want to manifest into your life. Your vision board should be full of words, phrases or photos of things that inspire you, but also things you aspire to create and see come to fruition in your life. By placing these images onto a board in an area that you will see them several times a day, you are bringing these dreams and plans into your thoughts more frequently. And what you think about, you bring about! Your vision board can also serve as a powerful reminder of the things you are working towards and motivate you to stay the course.

At first, I was hesitant to try to work with vision boards. A certain new friend was divinely placed in my life during a time when I was feeling stuck. She opened me up to a whole new way of thinking and introduced me to several books that would mark the beginning of my journey towards waking up to my potential. The first time my new friend shared with me the idea of creating a vision board, I was a little skeptical. The idea of putting my most intimate dreams and aspirations out for all to see made me feel a little too vulnerable. However, I decided I was willing to give just about anything a try because I knew I wanted to find my purpose and my current way of going about things was no longer serving me. Creating a vision board allowed me to finally admit things to myself about what I truly desired for my life and when I opened up to these new possibilities I knew the seeds had been planted – the seeds of hope for a future far brighter than I had ever previously imagined!

I became a true believer as I have started to see things from my vision board manifest one by one. Keep in mind that these things by no means happened overnight, but I have had faith that all of the desires of my heart are on their way in their perfect time. When focusing on your vision, hold space in your mind for the possibility that your vision could be limited and that something even better might be coming your way in its place. It is also essential to go back to your vision board from time to time and add and/or remove things as your dreams manifest or shift. Your vision board is an ever-evolving tool!

What you'll need:

- Large poster board (either cork or foam)
- A pair of scissors
- Push pins or glue/tape
- Magazines or printed images from photographs in your

own life

Instructions:

1. Setting an intention – Fill your board with words and images that make you feel strong, happy and empowered.
2. Find a space in your house or office where you can create the vision board and light candles, incense or put on soft music to set the tone of creating.
3. Prepare your working area and flip through magazines and images and select those that resonate with you. Focus on how the images make you feel.
4. Continue the process until you are satisfied with the layout and begin gluing, taping or pinning the images onto the board.
5. Spend time each day looking at the board to connect with what it would be like to live your dream life!

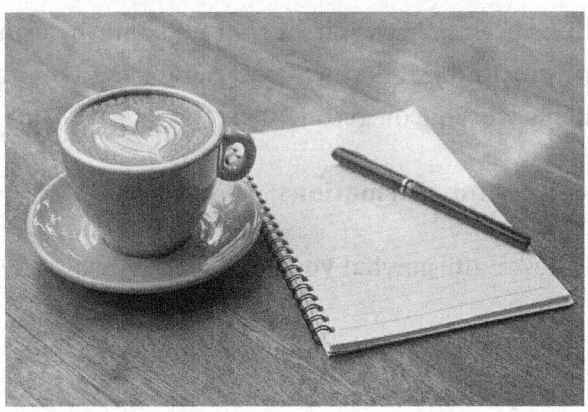

Affirmations

Affirmations are powerful grounding statements you make to focus your energy on positive outcomes. I remember when I was going through a tough transition in my life around age 25, I would say to myself, "I trust myself. I love myself." The brain cannot think a negative thought and a positive thought at the same time. Inserting two positive thoughts to negate a negative one is a simple way to start doing affirmations.

Affirmations can also create feelings of happiness, joy, appreciation, and gratitude that then, magnetize people, resources, and opportunities to come to you to help you achieve your goals. The idea of affirmations is to bombard the subconscious mind with positive thoughts to replace the many negative thought patterns that have evolved over time.

Michael Losier is an author who wrote a book titled, *"Law of Attraction: The Science of Attracting More of What You Want and Less of What You Don't Want."* In the book, he says that our brain will reject any thought that is not congruent with who we think we are. For example, if we think we are overweight and unhealthy, saying the affirmation *"I am healthy and thin"* will not register as a positive thought to our brain. We can change this dynamic by using the phrase, *"I am in the process of..."* that way we know we are not there yet, but we are actively working on getting there.

Some guidelines for affirmations:

1. Never affirm what you don't want. Always say what you do want.
2. Make affirmations for yourself only.
3. Be specific and concise.
4. Include an emotional word in the sentence.

Here are some other examples you may enjoy:

Self-Love:

1. Today I choose to release all that does not serve me and invite in self-compassion and love.
2. I am strong and empowered. I can do anything!
3. I am open to stepping into my power and experiencing life to the fullest.
4. I attract exactly what I need in each moment.
5. I love myself and honor myself for exactly who I am.
6. When my perspective changes, so does my reality.
7. I am good enough just as I am.

Health:

1. I am in the process of feeling more energy and vitality.
2. I am in the process of healing my mind, body, and spirit.
3. I nourish my body through the healthful food I eat.
4. I am in the process of feeling confident about the choices I make for my health.
5. I choose to treat my body with respect.

Finances:

1. I am in the process of becoming abundant and experience ease with my finances.
2. I feel safe and secure no matter what amount is in my bank account.
3. I trust that I am being taken care of and surrender my finances to a higher power.

How to use your affirmations:

1. Write out your affirmations on sticky notes and place them around your house – in your bedroom, on your bathroom mirror or in your car. Look at them daily.
2. Print out affirmation cards and laminate them. Read them daily as a part of your morning meditation practice.
3. Stating these affirmations out loud with enthusiasm magnifies the impact!
4. Write out the time of day you will review these affirmations.
5. Review and add new ones as you grow and expand!

I would also recommend listening to Louise Hay on YouTube or purchasing her CDs and audios. Louise has plenty of positive affirmation audios to listen to. These audios will add to your spiritual practice and facilitate healing of old negative belief systems.

Gratitude

Developing a daily gratitude practice can have positive results. By choosing to live each moment with an attitude of gratitude, you can change the way you see your world and live your life. In today's social media-crazed society, it is easier than ever to get into the poor habit of comparing yourself or your life to that of your friends or even to strangers. When we falsely perceive these posts as reality it can be tempting to feel like we aren't measuring up. Thoughts like "I'm not good enough," or "I don't have enough," "I'm not pretty enough or successful enough" and so on can subconsciously run in the background while we scroll through our feed. When we repeat this behavior multiple times a day, it's no wonder we think we don't have enough and that we would certainly be happier once we've received that thing that someone else has.

It is time to stop, reboot and get grateful! Experiencing gratitude is an important part of your journey toward awakening to your true potential and having a daily practice is an important tool to have in your spiritual tool belt. Choosing to focus your attention on all of the things you currently have in your life to be grateful for will inspire you, replacing feelings of lack that leave you wanting more.

Being in a state of gratitude encourages you to give yourself more love, acceptance, and appreciation for exactly where you are and what you have today. There are endless ways to incorporate a gratitude practice into your daily routine, and the best part is it's free, can be practiced from anywhere and doesn't require you to carve out huge amounts of time. Your gratitude practice should be unique to you and can be both a private practice and one that you can share with your loved ones!

If you love putting pen to paper and find journaling therapeutic, grab your journal and start simple. Start your morning each day by writing five things you are grateful for. It could be something as simple as your new favorite candle or your favorite pair of cozy socks. If you don't choose to keep a physical journal, there are endless amounts of free gratitude apps that you can download. These apps can provide you with a new writing prompt each day and send you a daily reminder, so you never forget to stop, reflect and experience gratitude!

Reframe how you view perceived unpleasant experiences by finding something to be grateful for. For example, maybe you have a long commute to and from work that you dread each day. Now think of at least two things you are grateful for when it comes to your commute. Maybe this is a time when you can have an uninterrupted phone call with your grandmother who is lonely. Or maybe this is the part of your day when you get to listen to your favorite podcast and enjoy your morning coffee. Complete this exercise as part of your daily practice for each situation that brings up feelings of contempt. By actively finding something to be grateful for, the next time you are experiencing feelings of not wanting to do this activity you can stop, reframe your thoughts and choose to experience gratitude instead. The more you practice gratitude, the easier it gets to reap its benefits!

You can also ask yourself, *"What was the best part of my day?"* This is a simple question that I ask myself every night before I fall asleep. By asking myself this question, it allows me to take an inventory of my day and think back to all of the things that brought me joy or appreciation. I almost always end up remembering something that may have seemed inconsequential at the moment, but upon reflection brings warmth to my heart. The more I practice this form of daily reflection, the better I have become at recognizing and feeling those feelings of gratitude in the present moment. When you choose an attitude of gratitude, you will naturally experience more joy in your life!

The more you practice feeling grateful for all of the ways that your life is abundant, the sooner you will begin to attract more things to be grateful for! As you bring self-awareness to your thoughts through your daily practice will begin to harness the power gratitude and awaken to your true potential.

Rhonda Byrne, author of *The Magic,* points out a passage from the Gospel of Matthew that states *"Whoever has will be given more, and he will have an abundance. Whoever does not have, even what he has will be taken from him."* According to Rhonda Byrne, there is a riddle hidden within this passage, and the answer to this riddle lies within one hidden word, and that word is gratitude. If you reread the passage and insert the word gratitude, the passage takes on a whole new light. *"Whoever has gratitude will be given more, and he will have an abundance. Whoever does not have gratitude, even what he has will be taken from him."*

In summary, here are three simple ways to start being grateful:

- Start a gratitude journal or download a gratitude app
- Reflect on the areas of your life that you may struggle with, reframe your thoughts, and find the ways you can experience it from a place a of gratitude
- Ask yourself: What was the best part of my day?

References

1. Schneider FW, Gruman JA, Coutts LM. Applied social psychology: Understanding and addressing social and practical problems. 2nd ed. Thousand Oaks, CA: Sage Publications, Inc; 2011.

2. Propst K. Self Sabotage & Goal Pursuit. The Diet Doc. thedietdoc.com/self-sabotage-goal-pursuit. Published May 30, 2014.

3. Grohol, John. 15 Common Cognitive Distortions. Psych Central. https://psychcentral.com/lib/15-common-cognitive-distortions/

4. "Difference between small and large intestine." Children's Hospital of Pittsburgh. UPMC. 2018. <http://www.chp.edu/our-services/transplant/intestine/education/about-small-large-intestines>.

5. Kerr M, Cafasso J. "Malabsorption syndrome." Healthline.com. 26 Sept 2015. <https://www.healthline.com/health/malabsorption>.

6. "Length of digestive tract." Viva health. 2018. Online. <https://www.vivahealth.org.uk/wheat-eaters-or-meat-eaters/length-digestive-tract>.

7. "The Enteric Nervous System: The Brain and the Gut." King's Psychology Network. <http://www.psyking.net/id36.htm>.

8. "Meditation Is Even More Powerful Than We Originally Thought." Huffington Post. 2014. Online. <https://www.huffingtonpost.com/2014/11/11/meditation-reduces-stress-harvard-study_n_6109404.html>

9. Thorpe, Matthew, MD, PhD "12 Science-Based Benefits of Meditation." 2017. Online. <https://www.healthline.com/nutrition/12-benefits-of-meditation>

10. Hawkins, David. Letting Go: The Pathway of Surrender. 2012. Hay House Inc.

11. Bray, George A et al. *The American Journal of Clinical Nutrition*, Volume 79, Issue 4, 1 April 2004, Pages 537–543,

https://doi.org/10.1093/ajcn/79.4.537.

12. Kirlian Photography.
http://www.energymedc.com/kirlian%20photography.htm

13. Bar-Yosef, R. et al. Halotherapy as asthma treatment in children: A randomized, controlled, prospective pilot study. Pediatr Pulmonol. 2017 May;52(5):580-587. doi: 10.1002/ppul.23621. Epub 2016 Oct 10.

14. H Lazarescu et al. Surveys on therapeutic effects of "halotherapy chamber with artificial salt-mine environment" on patients with certain chronic allergenic respiratory pathologies and infectious-inflammatory pathologies. J Med Life. 2014; 7(Spec Iss 2): 83–87.

15. Adams, Claire. Promoting Self-Compassionate Attitudes toward eating among restrictive and guilty eaters. Journal of Social and Clinical Psychology, Vol. 26, No. 10, 2007, pp. 1120–1144.

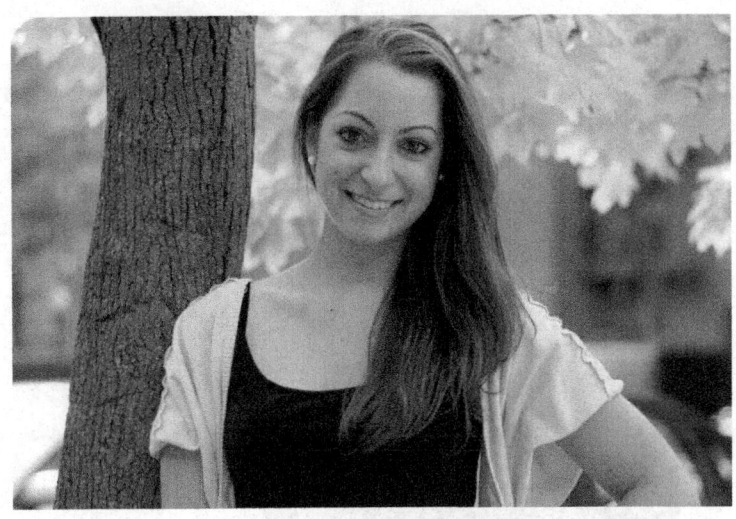

About the Author

Dr. Christina Tarantola, PharmD, CHC, CHt is a licensed pharmacist, certified health coach, certified hypnotherapist and Founder of Enlightened Wellness Solutions, a nutrition consulting company geared to empower people to take charge of their health!

For the last 6 years, Dr. Christina has been providing educational health talks in the NYC and Pittsburgh area, sharing her expertise on the monthly podcast segment on The Pharmacy Podcast, writing articles for Pharmacy Times and creating relevant, informative YouTube videos and newsletters to empower her clients to live healthy lives!

Dr. Christina's mission is to help reconnect people with the love, radiance, and energy within them. When you begin to connect with your "light", you naturally uncover your joy and fulfillment, which is what we all seek. This journey begins within and creates a powerful domino effect, ultimately making a positive impact on our world.

Contributors

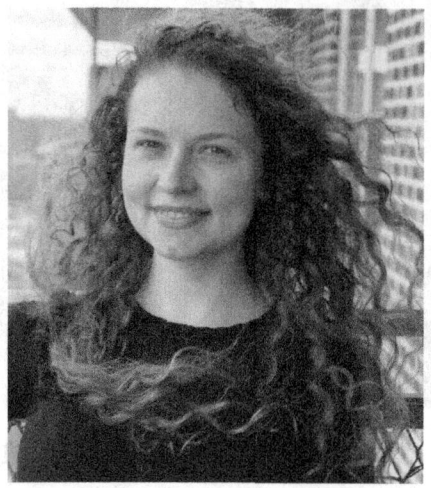

Marina Buksov (a.k.a. Dr. Marina Book at RawFork.com), is a registered Doctor of Pharmacy, Health Coach/Nutritionist, and lifelong learner of the healing arts. She is currently studying Clinical Herbalism at Arbor Vitae Traditional School of Herbalism in New York. Marina hopes to use her integrated background to educate and consult patients about the least invasive and most natural methods for healing the spirit-body-mind. When she is not studying, Marina likes to dance, paint, and make various concoctions such as tea blends, meals, DIY projects.

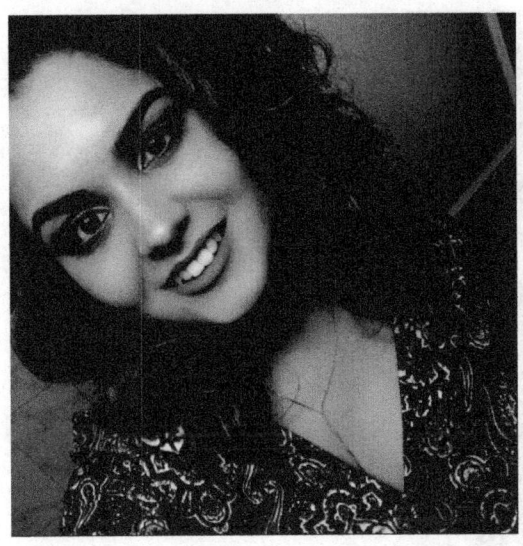

Dr. Nicole Zimmerman is a New York State licensed Doctor of Pharmacy. She has a passion for helping others, holistic and emotional healing, and the pharmacy profession. Through her own journey of self-healing, she developed a love for meditation, mindfulness, traditional Eastern medicine practices, and integrative nutrition, and shares what she researches and practices with others who are looking to heal themselves from the inside out. This year, she plans to become a certified health coach and jumpstart her own health consulting business to help pioneer the integration of pharmacy and preventative medicine.

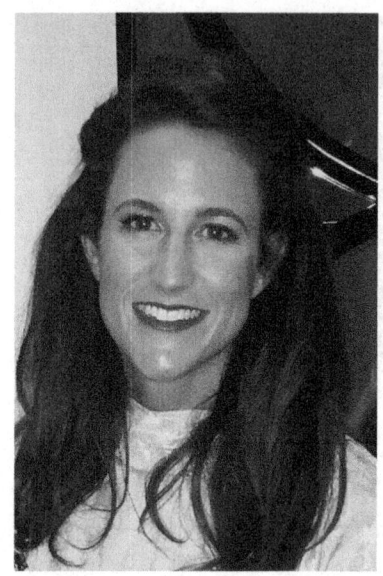

Krissy Hutinger obtained her Doctor of Pharmacy degree from the University of Missouri-Kansas City and has been a practicing community pharmacist for the last 6 years. She is currently enrolled at the Institute of Integrative Nutrition to become a certified health coach. To supplement her practice, she is developing a coaching business to educate patients on the role that nutrition and overall wellbeing play on disease prevention.

Krissy believes in a holistic approach to healing that integrates physical, emotional and social health. She believes pharmacists are uniquely positioned to help their patients become advocates of their own health and is excited to be among those who are leading the current healthcare system towards one that places an emphasis on preventative health measures.

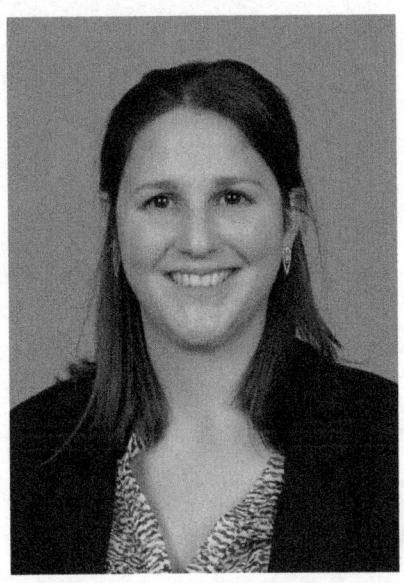

DawnDee Bostwick is a third-year pharmacy student at Northeast Ohio Medical University and will receive her Doctor of Pharmacy degree in May 2019. She believes healing starts with food, and good nutrition is the cornerstone in the prevention and treatment of diseases. She is a former journalist and holds degrees in journalism and English literature from the University of Oklahoma. DawnDee is a wife and mother, and a follower of Christ. When she's not involved with her studies, you'll find her preparing meals, spending time with her family, or reading.

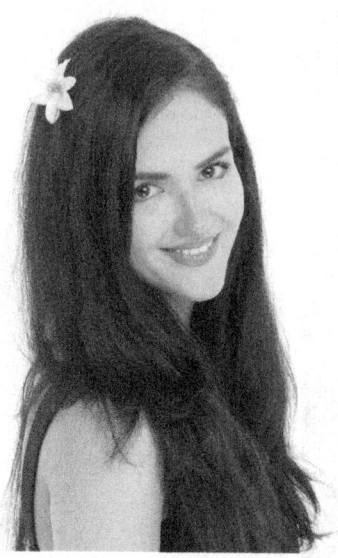

Niloufar Malekzadeh is a pharmacist from Vancouver, Canada who is passionate about preventative medicine and the mind/body connection, as well as helping people take simple steps every day to improve their health dramatically. Prior to pharmacy, she studied nutrition at the University of British Columbia and in her journey of self-growth and awareness, she discovered ways in which she could help others regain the power back in their lives by paying attention to "the little things". She hopes to enrich the lives of others by encouraging them to take charge of their health and well-being.

Made in the USA
Middletown, DE
15 November 2025

21141580R00099